Anaesthesia and the Practice of Medicine: Historical Perspectives

Anaesthesia and the Practice of Medicine: Historical Perspectives

Keith Sykes

with
John Bunker
Contributing Editor

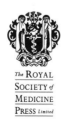

The ROYAL
SOCIETY of
MEDICINE
PRESS Limited

First published in Great Britain in 2007 by the Royal Society of Medicine Press Ltd, UK
Reprinted in 2011 by
Hodder Arnold, an imprint of Hodder Education, a division of Hachette UK
338 Euston Road, London NW1 3BH

http://www.hodderarnold.com

Hachette UK's policy is to use papers that are natural, renewable and recyclable products and made from wood grown in sustainable forests. The logging and manufacturing processes are expected to conform to the environmental regulations of the country of origin.

Whilst the advice and information in this book are believed to be true and accurate at the date of going to press, neither the author[s] nor the publisher can accept any legal responsibility or liability for any errors or omissions that may be made. In particular, (but without limiting the generality of the preceding disclaimer) every effort has been made to check drug dosages; however it is still possible that errors have been missed. Furthermore, dosage schedules are constantly being revised and new side-effects recognized. For these reasons the reader is strongly urged to consult the drug companies' printed instructions, and their websites, before administering any of the drugs recommended in this book.

British Library Cataloguing in Publication Data
A catalogue record for this book is available from the British Library

Library of Congress Cataloging-in-Publication Data
A catalog record for this book is available from the Library of Congress

ISBN-13   978-0-340-92958-2
3 4 5 6 7 8 9 10

The illustration on the cover shows an amputation being performed in the operating theatre of the old St Thomas' Hospital, London, before the introduction of general anaesthesia in 1846. The painting is by an anonymous artist and was discovered behind a plaster wall in a house in East Anglia. It is believed that it was painted between 1774–8. The original was stolen in 2001. It is reproduced by kind permission of the Royal College of Surgeons of England and the Curator of the Old Operating Theatre, Museum and Herb Garrett, London.

The logo of the Royal Society of Medicine is a registered trade mark and is used by Hodder & Stoughton Ltd under licence.

Typeset in 9.5 on 11pt Times by Phoenix Photosetting, Chatham, Kent

What do you think about this book? Or any other Hodder Arnold title?
Please visit our website: www.hodderarnold.com

Contents

Part 1: Anaesthesia: the first 100 years

Although the soporific effects of ether had been described in 1540, surgeons continued to operate on the conscious patient for a further 300 years. When anaesthesia finally arrived, it did so as an offshoot of the recreational drug culture of the time, and with the leading players contesting their role in its discovery.

On 11 September 1884, a 27-year old surgeon in Vienna, Carl Koller, operated on a patient with glaucoma, having anaesthetized the eye with an aqueous solution of cocaine. It was the first recorded administration of a local anaesthetic, and led to a new era in surgery. Others, possibly including Sigmund Freud, had noted the benumbing effects of cocaine, and had even suggested its possible use in surgery, but it was Koller who demonstrated its feasibility.

For general anaesthesia to progress in the 20th century, it was necessary to develop an apparatus that could deliver known concentrations of anaesthetic gases and vapours to a leak-proof breathing system. The anaesthetist then had to learn how to ventilate the lungs artificially and to prevent their collapse when the surgeon entered the chest. The development of tracheal tubes with an inflatable cuff provided a secure airway that enabled the anaesthetist to control ventilation, so opening the door for thoracic surgery and the later introduction of curare.

Part 2: Professionalism in anaesthesia: the reluctant universities and the Second World War

Part 3: New horizons: the scientific background of anaesthesia and the emergence of intensive care

Part 4: The relief of pain in childbirth and the care of the newborn

Part 5: Anaesthesia yesterday, today and tomorrow

During the last half-century, anaesthesia has been responsible for major changes in medical practice, and has become a scientific discipline in its own right. Today, anaesthesia is one of the largest specialities in the UK National Health Service, but it faces two major problems: the impact of the European Working Time Directive on clinical services and training, and the erosion of the academic base that is essential for the future development of the subject.

Biographical notes

Keith Sykes: Born in England 1925. Medical education at Magdalene College, Cambridge 1944–46, and University College Hospital (UCH), London 1946–49. House physician and surgeon posts at UCH and Norfolk and Norwich Hospitals 1949–50, followed by service in the Royal Army Medical Corps, British Army of the Rhine 1950–52. Anaesthetic training at UCH 1952–58, with one-year Fellowship in Anesthesia at Massachusetts General Hospital, Boston 1954–55. Extensive travel within the USA and Canada funded by a Rickman Godlee Travelling Scholarship, UCH Medical School. Appointed Lecturer in Anaesthesia and Consultant Anaesthetist at the Postgraduate Medical School and the Hammersmith Hospital, London 1958, Clinical Reader 1967–70 and Professor of Clinical Anaesthesia 1970–80. Nuffield Professor of Anaesthetics, and Fellow, Pembroke College, University of Oxford 1980–91. Honorary Fellow, Pembroke College, Oxford 1996. Consultant Adviser in Anaesthetics to the Chief Medical Officer, Department of Health and Social Security 1986–92. Knight Bachelor 1991. Extensive overseas lecture tours to USA, South America, Australasia, South Africa, Far East and Europe, and author of papers and books on respiratory failure, clinical measurement and monitoring, and respiratory problems in intensive care.

John P Bunker: Graduated from Harvard University College and Medical School, and trained in anaesthesia at George Washington School of Medicine and at the Massachusetts General Hospital, Boston. Was on the Anesthesia Faculty at Harvard University from 1950 to 1960, and at Stanford University from 1960 to 1989, where he was Chairman of the Department of Anesthesia from 1960 to 1972. Visiting Professor of Preventive and Social Medicine, Harvard Medical School 1973–75. Acting Director, Center for the Analysis of Health Practices, Harvard School of Public Health 1974–75. Professor of Family, Community and Preventive Medicine, Stanford University School of Medicine 1976–88.

He has held visiting professorships at Harvard Medical School, Harvard School of Public Health, Westminster Hospital Medical School, London and University College London Medical School. He is a recipient of Fellowships from the National Institutes of Health, the Commonwealth Fund, the John Simon Guggenheim Foundation and the Henry J Kaiser Foundation. He is an author and editor of books on anaesthesia, surgery and health policy.

Preface

In June 2000, John Bunker and I met by chance in the library of the Royal Society of Medicine in London. John had been Henry K Beecher's First Assistant when I spent a year at the Massachusetts General Hospital, Boston in 1954–55 and had supervised my research project that compared ether anaesthesia with the new technique of anaesthesia using muscle relaxant drugs. As we chatted, he expressed concern that the contributions of anaesthesia to medicine were being forgotten. Would I care to join him in an attempt to set the record straight? Since I had utilized this topic when lecturing to non-medical audiences, I offered him my notes. He felt that our joint experience could yield an interesting story, and we agreed to cooperate on a book that would have a transatlantic approach.

Shortly before I retired in 1991, I was asked to give the Griffith Lecture at the 1992 World Congress of Anaesthesiology, so I began to study the history of 'curare', the South American Indian arrow poison that Harold Griffith had first used to produce muscular relaxation during anaesthesia in 1942. The story of curare proved fascinating, but the research made me realize what an enormous impact the intravenous anaesthetic drugs and curare had made on both anaesthesia and surgery.

Before curare, patients had to suffer the choking sensation, pounding in the head, disorientation and frightening dreams associated with the inhalation of the highly irritant vapour of ether or chloroform; they were then likely to suffer prolonged nausea and vomiting when consciousness returned. With ether, the inhalation often had to be continued for 30–45 minutes before the abdominal muscles relaxed enough to allow intra-abdominal surgery, and the deep anaesthesia not only caused respiratory and circulatory depression, but also resulted in a prolonged delay in the recovery of consciousness. By contrast, an intravenous induction with thiopental and curare, followed by light anaesthesia with nitrous oxide and oxygen, provided perfect operating conditions within a few minutes, with minimal side-effects and a rapid recovery. It is small wonder that surgeons exploited this new technique by developing new operations and by operating on patients who might have succumbed if they had been anaesthetized with the older agents.

As I began to write, I realized that I had been privileged to participate in many of the developments that I was describing. I had worked in the ward crammed with 30 or so 'iron lungs' during the Boston poliomyelitis epidemic of 1955, but I was unable to utilize the techniques developed in the 1952 Copenhagen epidemic because there was no suitable ventilator in the hospital. In 1959, Professor EB Adams invited me to set up a respiratory unit in Durban, South Africa, where we were able to conduct a controlled trial that showed that total paralysis with curare, with breathing supported by a mechanical ventilator, could halve the mortality from neonatal tetanus. In 1961, I was able to introduce the use of mechanical ventilators to support patients with other types of respiratory failure and so to develop the Intensive Care Unit at the Royal Postgraduate Medical School and Hammersmith Hospital in West London. During my 22 years of practice in that exciting, research-orientated institution, I helped to provide anaesthesia for the first patients to undergo open-heart surgery in the UK and to set up the first UK in-hospital resuscitation service. During this period, we were able to attract many research workers from the UK and abroad and in 1970, with the continued support of the Head of Department, Professor (now Sir Gordon) Robson, I was made Professor of Clinical Anaesthesia.

John Bunker recognized the significance of these events and encouraged me to insert some personal reminiscences into the text; I responded by asking him to write his story of the National Halothane Study and to collaborate on the chapters on the history of general and local anaesthesia, pain, obstetric analgesia, patient safety, and Virginia Apgar's contribution to perinatology. Working together, and editing each other's contributions, we gradually built up a story that tells how skills that were developed in the operating room have been increasingly applied to problems in other branches of medical practice. It has been an exciting and rewarding experience.

KEITH SYKES

Acknowledgements

We would like to thank Dr Julian Tudor Hart, Professor HP Lambert and the late Dr JSM Zorab for reading the late draft of the book and providing invaluable comments. Thanks are also due to Patrick Sim, Librarian of the Wood Library–Museum of Anesthesiology of the American Society of Anesthesiologists, Trish Willis and Iris Boening of the Anaesthesia Heritage Centre of the Association of Anaesthetists of Great Britain and Ireland, Professor RJ Kitz of Harvard Medical School, and other colleagues for advice and help in obtaining illustrations, the sources of which are acknowledged in the figure captions. Parts of the text were read by members of our families, and by our wives Michelle Sykes and Lavinia Loughridge, and to them we express our gratitude for their advice, understanding and patience throughout the six-year gestation period of this book. We accept full responsibility for any errors and omissions and acknowledge the help provided by staff of the Royal Society of Medicine Press.

Introduction

By the end of 1846, the clinical efficacy of ether anaesthesia for operative surgery had been demonstrated both in Boston and in London. In 1847, chloroform was shown to be an even more potent general anaesthetic. The techniques for the administration of these drugs were primitive (but so also were those of surgery), and they remained so for the rest of the century. The early anaesthetists were general practitioners, medical students, nurses or other untrained personnel, and their responsibilities were limited to rendering the surgical patient unconscious and immobile.

Today's anaesthetists are highly trained clinicians. Their primary responsibilities are still the provision of anaesthesia and pre- and postoperative care for surgical patients, but about a quarter of their clinical work lies outside the operating theatre environment: in the administration and day-to-day care in intensive care units, in the diagnosis and treatment of chronic pain, in providing analgesia and anaesthesia in obstetrics and for day care surgery, and, perhaps most importantly, in providing a 24-hour call service for the Accident and Emergency Department. The advances in anaesthesia that have occurred, and how they have become incorporated into mainstream medicine, are recounted in the pages that follow. Since the setting is transatlantic, some differences in terminology need to be addressed.

Although the UK and USA share a common language, the method of practice and the terminology differ significantly. The word *anaesthesia* is of Greek origin and simply means 'without pain'. Its use to describe the process of pain relief during surgery or dentistry is attributed to Oliver Wendell Holmes, physician, poet and humorist notable for his medical research and teaching, and for the 'Breakfast Table' series of essays. In the UK, anaesthesia has nearly always been administered by doctors or medical students, and the person who gives the anaesthetic is called an *anaesthetist*. In the USA, prior to the Second World War, anaesthesia was administered primarily by nurses and other medical personnel, but rarely by doctors. Those doctors who did specialize in anaesthesia were called *physician–anesthetists* to distinguish them from *nurse–anesthetists*. As anaesthesia approached maturity shortly before the Second World War, the American physicians changed their name to *anesthesiologist* to indicate that they were medically qualified doctors and not nurses. British spelling and terminology will be used throughout except when the topic has a direct American connotation.

Both Keith Sykes and John Bunker are anaesthetists who have worked in the Massachusetts General Hospital in Boston, Massachusetts, and in University College Hospital, London – the two hospitals where the first general anaesthetics for surgery were given in 1846. Our professional careers spanned a 50-year period of advances in anaesthesia, from the days when ether was considered to be the only safe anaesthetic to the era of sophisticated anaesthetic techniques that are practised today. Both of us were privileged to play a part in some of the advances described in this book. We were involved in the debates over the safety of the new muscle relaxant drug 'curare' introduced in 1942, and over the safety of the new inhalation agent halothane, introduced in 1956; we were first-hand witnesses of Beecher's attempts to quantify pain and assess the efficacy of pain-relieving drugs following the Second World War. We participated in the development of intensive care units that resulted directly from Bjørn Ibsen's successful application of the anaesthetist's techniques for providing artificial ventilation in the Copenhagen poliomyelitis epidemic of 1952. Both of us were privileged to have practised in a golden age in which anaesthesia grew from a technical speciality to become part of the practice of medicine.

To set the story in perspective, we have gone back to the beginning. Since general anaesthesia had its origins in the recreational drug culture of the time, we take the reader back to the 'laughing gas parties' and 'ether frolics' of the early 19th century, and we then trace the evolution of anaesthesia from the earliest times to the present day. It is an intriguing tale.

Part 1

Anaesthesia: The first 100 years

In 1900, Sir Frederick Treves, the surgeon who later removed the appendix of King Edward VII two days before his planned Coronation, addressed the Annual Meeting of the British Medical Association in Ipswich and made these comments about the introduction of anaesthesia:

'The changes that the discovery has wrought in the personality of the surgeon, in his bearing, in his methods, and in his capabilities are as wondrous as the discovery itself. The operator is undisturbed by the harass of alarms and the misery of giving pain. He can afford to be leisurely without fear of being regarded as timorous. To the older surgeon every tick of the clock upon the wall was a mandate for haste, every groan of the patient a call for hurried action, and he alone did best who had the quickest fingers and the hardest heart. Time now counts for little, and success is no longer to be measured by the beatings of a watch. The mask of the anaesthetist has blotted out the anguished face of the patient, and the horror of a vivisection on a fellow-man has passed away. Thus it happens that the surgeon has gained dignity, calmness, confidence, and, not least of all, the gentle hand.

Anaesthetics have, moreover, greatly extended the domain of surgery by rendering possible operations which before could only have been dreamt about, and by allowing elaborate measures to be carried out step by step.

The introduction of anaesthetics has not only developed surgery, but it has engendered surgeons. It has opened up the craft to many, for in the pre-anaesthetic days the qualities required for success in operating were qualities to be expected only in the few.'

(Treves F. Address in surgery: the surgeon in the nineteenth century. *British Medical Journal* 1900;**ii**:284–9)

1 In the beginning

Although the soporific effects of ether had been described in 1540, surgeons continued to operate on the conscious patient for a further 300 years. When anaesthesia finally arrived, it did so as an offshoot of the recreational drug culture of the time, and with the leading players hotly contesting their role in its discovery.

Surgery before anaesthesia

On the 30 September 1811, some 35 years before the demonstration that anaesthesia could abolish the pain of a surgical operation, Napoleon's Surgeon-in-Chief, Dominique-Jean Larrey, removed the cancerous breast of the novelist Fanny Burney. She later wrote a long and harrowing account of the operation. After describing how she had lain on a mattress and had refused to be held down by the seven men and the nurse attending the procedure, she wrote:

'Yet, when the dreadful steel was plunged into my breast – cutting through veins–arteries–flesh–nerves – I needed no injunctions not to restrain my cries. I began a scream that lasted unintermittingly during the whole time of the incision – & I almost marvel that it rings not in my ears still! so excruciating was the agony. When the wound was made & the instrument was withdrawn, the pain seemed undiminished, for the air that suddenly rushed into those delicate parts felt like a mass of minute but sharp and forked poinards, that were tearing the edges of the wound, – but when again I felt the instrument – describing a curve – cutting against the grain, if I may so say, while the flesh resisted in a manner so forcible as to oppose & tire the hand of the operator, who was forced to change from the right hand to the left – then, indeed, I thought I must have expired, I attempted no more to open my eyes, they felt as if hermetically shut, & so firmly closed, that the Eyelids seemed indented into the Cheeks'.[1]

The excruciating pain felt by Fanny Burney was experienced by all the patients who were forced to have an operation at that time. And yet, 11 years previously, the young scientist Humphry Davy had described the pain-relieving properties of nitrous oxide (see below). Why, then, was the gas not used to relieve the pain of surgery until 1844? Was it the fear of the unconscious state, the fear of the outcome, or a reluctance to interfere with nature? Perhaps, it was all three. But we must remember that in those days there were no cures for disease, early death was common, working conditions were harsh, and most aspects of life were generally uncomfortable, so pain was accepted as a part of life. There were no pain-relieving drugs other than laudanum (an alcoholic extract of opium), and almost everyone suffered toothache or some other type of pain at some time in their life. There was also biblical support for the belief that pain was a necessary part of the human condition.

It is true that there had been some attempts to relieve the pain associated with surgery. The 1st century AD physician Dioscorides administered the root of the mandragora plant boiled in wine in an attempt to diminish the pain of surgery.[2] Later, some surgeons attempted to abolish pain by compressing the nerve or blood vessels supplying a limb, while military surgeons noted that extreme cold diminished the pain of an amputation on the battlefield. Although there are a number of reports of the administration of pain-relieving drugs such as hemp, hemlock or laudanum, the effects must have been variable because of the inability to standardize the dose: a drug powerful enough to produce unconsciousness could just as easily produce death. Other patients were given alcohol, but this was more commonly used to relieve pain after the operation, particularly in military surgery. Undoubtedly, the prospect of pain was a strong deterrent to the practice of surgery, so very few operations were performed, but, when the operation was potentially life-saving, the patient had to submit to the knife and hope that the surgeon would operate as quickly as possible.

Pneumatic medicine

In 1772, Joseph Priestley, a dissenting clergyman, political theorist and experimental scientist, discovered the gas nitrous oxide (N_2O), but at that time no one conceived that it would be used to produce anaesthesia. Later, he and Carl Wilhelm Scheele, a Swedish chemist, identified another gas that the French chemist Antoine-Laurent Lavoisier subsequently named oxygen (O_2). It was soon realized that oxygen was taken up by the lungs and that carbon dioxide (CO_2) was given out, so it is not surprising that Priestley should have urged physicians to explore the possibility of inhaling other gases as a treatment for respiratory diseases such as tuberculosis, which was rampant at that time. The idea was taken up by Thomas Beddoes, an Oxford physician and chemist who, in 1794, set up the Medical Pneumatic Institution in Bristol to further these aims.[3,4] Beddoes was acquainted with members of the Birmingham Lunar Society (who held meetings at the time of the full moon to allow members to see their way home). Josiah Wedgwood, one of its prominent members, made a large donation in support of the Institution, while another member, James Watt, inventor of the steam engine, designed and constructed some of the apparatus used to manufacture and store the gases.

In 1798, Beddoes met the 19-year-old Humphry Davy, who had been carrying out experiments with nitrous oxide in the small town of Penzance, Cornwall. He was so impressed by Davy's accomplishments that he appointed him Medical Superintendent of the Pneumatic Institution. While examining the properties of nitrous oxide in Bristol, Davy found that inhalation of a few breaths of the gas relieved the pain caused by an acute infection in his gums. He also noted that the inhalation of nitrous oxide produced strange but pleasurable sensations, excitement, and intoxicating behaviour, often accompanied by irrational peals of laughter. Two of Beddoes' acquaintances, the poets Robert Southey and Samuel Taylor Coleridge, were among those who enjoyed the effects of Davy's 'laughing gas'. In his *Researches, Chemical and Philosophical: Chiefly Concerning Nitrous Oxide*, published in 1800, Davy wrote:

> *'As nitrous oxide in its extensive operation appears capable of destroying physical pain, it may probably be used with advantage during surgical operations in which no great effusion of blood takes place'.[5]*

Davy had been apprenticed to a surgeon in Penzance, so it is surprising that neither he nor those of his colleagues who also inhaled nitrous oxide followed up this suggestion. This may seem strange to us today, but Davy was primarily interested in chemical research. It must also be remembered that attitudes to pain were very different in the 18th century; patients expected pain and tolerated it because there was no known way of abolishing it. But, as the anaesthetist W Stanley Sykes commented in 1960:

> *'What is surprising is that his suggestion was ignored by the very people whom it should have interested most: that surgeons should have continued for nearly fifty years longer to operate on screaming, struggling patients in full consciousness. Surely a lasting testimonial to their thickheadedness'.[6]*

The first attempt to produce pain-free surgery: Henry Hill Hickman

In fact, it was carbon dioxide, and not nitrous oxide, that was the first gas to be used in an attempt to produce surgical anaesthesia. The investigator was Henry Hill Hickman, a general practitioner in Ludlow in Shropshire. He was born in 1800, the year that Davy first suggested that nitrous oxide might be used for the relief of pain during surgery, and when he started to practise medicine he became concerned about the pain felt by patients when he had to perform surgical procedures. Hickman knew that carbon dioxide was present in expired gas and that it was produced during the fermentation of beer. In February 1824, he wrote a letter to TA Knight, a Fellow of the Royal Society who lived nearby, and described seven experiments in which he claimed that he had carried out painless surgical procedures on animals while they inhaled the gas. In August of that year, he published a pamphlet in which he set out in more detail his proposal that the inhalation of carbon dioxide should be used to relieve the pain of surgical operations. In the pamphlet, he stated:

> *'I feel perfectly satisfied that any surgical operation might be performed with quite as much safety upon a subject in an insensible state as in a sensible state, and that a patient might be kept with perfect safety long enough in an insensible state, for the performance of the most tedious operation. . . . I believe that there are few, if any Surgeons, who could not operate more skilfully when they were conscious they were not inflicting pain'.*[7]

Unfortunately, Knight seems to have been more interested in the growth of trees than in Hickman's proposals, and it is not clear whether Hickman's ideas were ever communicated to other members of the scientific community. In 1828, Hickman decided to try and further his aims by travelling to Paris, then the recognized centre of scientific research. In desperation, Hickman wrote to Charles X of France, and, in 1829, a committee was set up to consider his claims. Only Napoleon's surgeon, Baron Larrey, who had operated on Fanny Burney, showed any interest, and in the following year Hickman died at the age of 30. It is now known that an excess of carbon dioxide in the blood can produce narcosis, but the side-effects would have precluded its use as an anaesthetic.[8]

The first administrations of an anaesthetic for surgery

Perhaps it is not surprising that anaesthesia should have finally been introduced by a dentist, for a dentist could only prosper if he succeeded in persuading the patient to tolerate the pain of a tooth extraction. It was, however, the recreational drug culture of the time that provided the stimulus for the final development of anaesthesia. In the 1820s and 1830s, a number of entrepreneurs provided public and private demonstrations of the exhilarating effects of 'laughing gas' both in the UK and in the USA (Figure 1.1). The inhalation of ether, a volatile liquid that had been synthesized in 1540 by the German botanist Valerius Cordus, produced similar effects and was used to enliven parties known as 'ether frolicks'. The intoxicating behaviour often resulted in minor injuries that were not noticed by the subjects until they returned to sobriety, so duplicating Davy's observation of pain relief during the inhalation of nitrous oxide.

Gardner Q Colton, Horace Wells and nitrous oxide (the 'laughing gas')

On the evening of 10 December 1844, an itinerant chemist, Gardner Q Colton, gave a demonstration of the exhilarating effects of nitrous oxide in Hartford, Connecticut. A dentist in the audience, Horace Wells, noted that one of the subjects had banged his shin during the inhalation but had not felt pain. Wells arranged for Colton to give a private demonstration of the effects of nitrous oxide the next day. Wells had been suffering from pain in a wisdom tooth and was so impressed by the demonstration that he asked Colton to administer nitrous oxide while the tooth was extracted. When Wells recovered consciousness, he realized the great potential of this new technique and proclaimed *'A new era in tooth-pulling'.*[9]

Colton taught Wells how to prepare the gas, and in the next month Wells used it for 15 dental extractions. The technique was simple: the nostrils were compressed and the gas was inhaled from an animal bladder through a wooden tube inserted into the mouth. When the patient became unconscious, the bag was removed and the tooth extracted. Since there was no air or oxygen in the bag, the patient would have died from lack of oxygen if the inhalation had been prolonged. Fortunately, the bag usually fell to the ground when the patient became unconscious, so allowing air to enter the lungs.

Later, Wells travelled to Boston where his old pupil and partner, William Thomas Green Morton (see below), introduced him to surgeons at the Massachusetts General Hospital. Wells had continued to experiment with the gas, and in 1845 he was invited to demonstrate the use of nitrous oxide to students in the Medical School. Unfortunately, the patient was not adequately anaesthetized and cried out as the tooth was

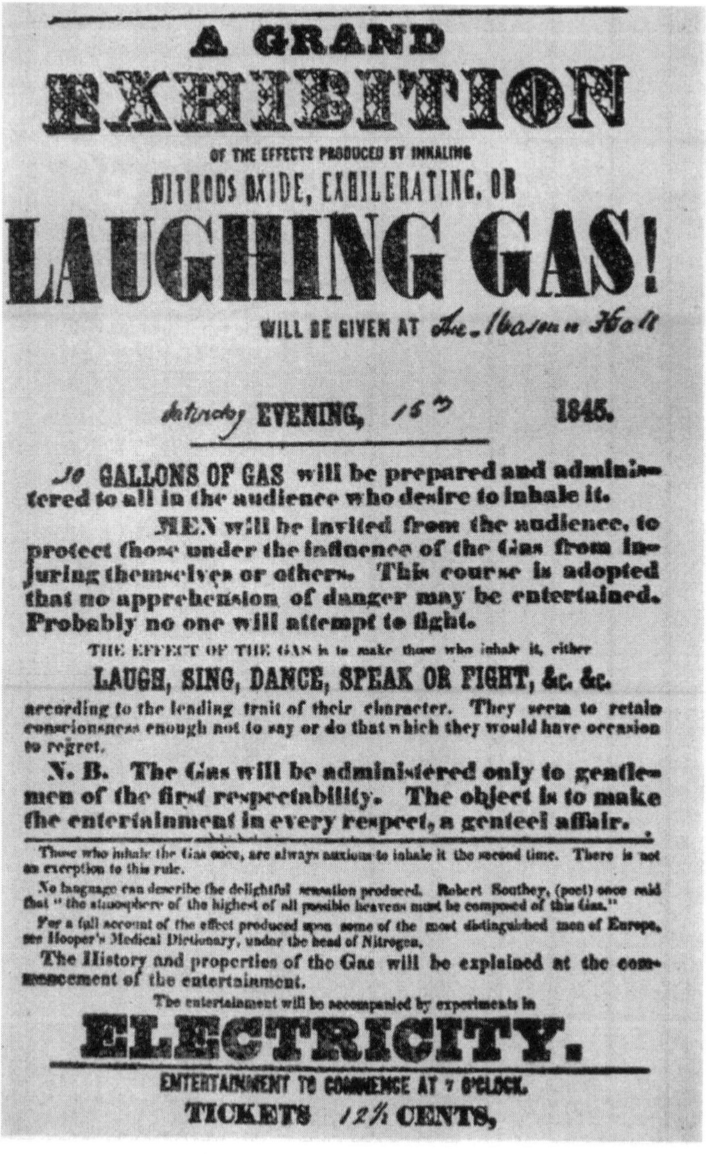

Figure 1.1 Playbill advertising a demonstration of the effects of nitrous oxide in 1845. (Reproduced with kind permission from the Association of Anaesthetists of Great Britain and Ireland.)

extracted. Wells was dismissed as a charlatan. He became depressed, later became addicted to chloroform, was sent to gaol for throwing sulphuric acid at a prostitute, and there committed suicide.[10]

Crawford W Long, William E Clarke, Charles T Jackson, William Thomas Green Morton and the battle for priority

Although Wells obviously played a key role in the early development of anaesthesia, there were two others who have a claim to priority. The first was William E Clarke, a medical student who lived in Rochester, New York. He frequently entertained his fellow students with inhalations of ether, and, in January 1842, he administered ether to a young woman called Miss Hobbie while a dentist, Elijah Pope, extracted a tooth. The second was Crawford Williamson Long, a general practitioner in Jefferson, Georgia. He described how he had witnessed the lack of pain felt by those who injured themselves when participating in ether frolics, and claimed that he had been the first person to put the observation to practical use by administering ether for a surgical operation on 30 March 1842. He gave ether to several other patients over the next few years, but did not report these cases until 1849, so the other pioneers did not know of his discovery.[11]

Because of the delay in the reporting of these early cases, it is generally accepted that it was the successful public administration of an ether anaesthetic by the dentist William Thomas Green Morton in 1846 that finally convinced the medical profession that anaesthesia could relieve the pain of surgery. Just as Gardner Q Colton played a key role in the introduction of nitrous oxide as an anaesthetic agent, so Charles T Jackson, a graduate of Harvard Medical School, pioneer chemist, geologist and mineralogist, played an equally indispensable role in facilitating Morton's successful demonstration of surgical anaesthesia. Wells had not been searching for an anaesthetic agent, but had recognized the useful properties of nitrous oxide during Colton's demonstration. Morton was searching for a drug to relieve the pain of dentistry, and it was Jackson who alerted him to the possible use of diethyl ether.

Morton knew of the failure of Wells to demonstrate the anaesthetic properties of nitrous oxide and so sought an agent of greater potency. He was familiar with the numbing effects of diethyl ether applied locally to the gums. Eager to investigate the possibility that it might produce relief of pain if inhaled, he was advised to seek the advice of Dr Jackson, whose classes he had attended at Harvard Medical School.[12] Morton was reluctant to do so, having heard of Jackson's bitter dispute with Samuel

Morse over credit for the invention of the electric telegraph and the signalling system later known as the Morse Code.*

Although he feared that he might suffer the same fate, Morton needed help and reluctantly sought it from Jackson. Morton and Jackson were playing a cat-and-mouse game. Morton was eager to have access to Jackson's chemical knowledge of ether but preferred to let Jackson think that he intended to use nitrous oxide. Jackson for his part believed that ether was the better agent, but he was cautious, worried that if Morton failed, he himself might be associated with the failure. In the event, Jackson did recommend the trial of ether, and Morton and two of his dental assistants went away to experiment on themselves. With further advice from Jackson that he should use purified rather than the impure commercial ether, Morton sought an opportunity to test its use in a patient.

The opportunity presented itself on 30 September 1846, and met with success. On the following day, the *Boston Journal* reported:

> *'Last evening, as we were informed by a gentleman who witnessed the operation, an ulcerated tooth was extracted from the mouth of an individual, without giving him the slightest pain. He was put into a kind of sleep, by inhaling a preparation, the effects of which lasted about three-quarters of a minute, just long enough to extract the tooth'.*[13]

The report came to the attention of Henry Jacob Bigelow, a surgeon at the Massachusetts General Hospital. Bigelow was sufficiently impressed to invite Morton to demonstrate its use in surgery at the hospital, despite Wells' failed demonstration with nitrous oxide the previous year. The operation took place on 16 October 1846 in what is now known as the ether dome in the Bullfinch building (Figure 1.2).

The surgeon was Professor John Collins Warren and the patient Edward Gilbert Abbott. The operation was for the excision of a congenital tumour in the neck. Morton had to make some last minute adjustments to his inhaler and was late for the appointment, so Warren prepared to begin surgery on the conscious patient. At the last minute, Morton rushed in and induced anaesthesia with a hastily devised glass

---

* Jackson and Morse, travelling from Le Havre to New York in 1832, had become acquainted and had discussed the future possibilities of electricity. Morse went on to develop and perfect his invention, for which he was handsomely rewarded by the US Congress. Morse was then astonished to read in a Boston newspaper that *'the discovery of the electro-magnetic telegraph, which S.F.B.Morse of New York claims to have made, was really made by our fellow-citizen Charles T. Jackson'*. Jackson pursued his claim, and it was seven years before Morse could shake off his pursuer.

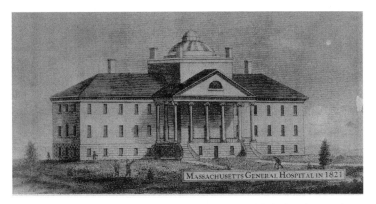

Figure 1.2 The Massachusetts General Hospital in 1821. At this time, patients could access the hospital from the Charles River behind the Bullfinch building. The operating theatre, later known as the ether dome, is in the centre of the building. (Reproduced with kind permission from the Wood Library–Museum of Anaesthesiology, Park Ridge, Illinois.)

inhaler that contained a sea sponge soaked with ether (Figure 1.3). Warren recounted what then transpired as follows:

'On October 17th [it was, in fact the 16th], *the patient being prepared for the operation, the apparatus was applied to his mouth by Dr. Morton for about three minutes, at the end of such time he sank into a state of insensibility. I immediately made an incision about three inches long through the skin of the neck, and began a dissection among important nerves and blood vessels without any expression of pain on the part of the patient. Soon after he began to speak incoherently, and appeared to be in an agitated state during the remainder of the operation. Immediately afterwards when he was asked whether he had suffered much, he said that he had felt as if his neck had been scratched; but subsequently, when I queried him on his feeling, his statement was that he did not experience pain at any time, although aware that the operation was proceeding'.*[14]

At the conclusion of the operation, Warren turned to the doctors and students and uttered the words that became famous throughout the medical world: *'Gentlemen, this is no humbug'.*

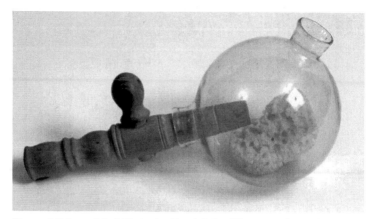

Figure 1.3 A model of Morton's ether inhaler. Ether was dropped onto the sponge and the vapour breathed through the wooden mouthpiece. (Nuffield Department of Anaesthetics, Oxford.)

Morton then tried to capitalize on his success by applying for a patent. He attempted to conceal the identity of the ether by calling it Letheon (from *Lethe*, the river in Hades, the waters of which, when imbibed, were supposed to produced amnesia), and he claimed sole credit for the discovery of anaesthesia. Jackson had provided essential advice, including the recommendation that Morton use 'pure' rather than commercial ether – advice that was instrumental in the successful demonstration – but Jackson initially distanced himself from any association with the outcome. When, in the event, ether anaesthesia became an instant success, Jackson proclaimed himself the true discoverer. Morton agreed to share patent profits with him, but the patent application was denied.

Morton became a national hero and the US Congress prepared to grant him an award of $100 000. Jackson, outraged at this turn of events, was able to delay Congressional approval, and ultimately to block it entirely. Jackson spent the remainder of his life attempting to blacken Morton's name and to promote his own. While Jackson failed in his claim as the discoverer of anaesthesia, his contribution was an essential one. Although Morton was deemed the sole discoverer of anaesthesia, there was ample credit for Jackson and Wells, as well as for Morton, and even for the reclusive Crawford Long.

Following Morton's death in 1868, Jackson continued to defame his character and professional stature. He was obsessed with the effort to claim sole credit as the discoverer of anaesthesia and to expunge Morton's name from human memory. As Morton's fame continued to mount and his own stature diminish, Jackson sank into depression and drink. That he had finally lost the battle, Jackson only fully realized some years later. Rene Fülöp-Miller describes the final blow as follows: Jackson had been strolling among the gardens and tombstones in Mt Auburn Cemetery in Cambridge when:

'... he suddenly caught sight of an aspiring monument – Morton's! What had led him hither? He could not tell. His brain was clouded by a long succession of sleepless nights and by the effects of the whisky in which he had indulged throughout the years since Morton's death. Standing before the monument he read the chiselled inscription: "William T.G.Morton, Inventor and Revealer of Anesthetic inhalation. By whom pain in surgery was averted and annulled. Before whom in all time surgery was agony. Since whom Science has control of Pain"'.[15] (Figure 1.4)*

Jackson started to scream, lost his reason, needed to be subdued and was institutionalized in the McLean Asylum nearby, where he remained until his death seven years later.[15] The epitaph on Jackson's tombstone would surely have satisfied his ego (Figure 1.5).

The news travels across the Atlantic

Following Morton's successful demonstration in October 1846, the news from Boston soon spread around the world via steamship mail. It has been claimed that the first ether anaesthetic in Europe was administered in the Dumfries and Galloway Royal Infirmary, Scotland on 19 December 1846, but the evidence is conflicting. On the same day, Frances Boot, an American physician practising in Gower Street, London, received news of the Boston anaesthetic. Boot immediately encouraged the dentist James Robinson to give a female patient ether for the extraction of a molar tooth. Boot was so impressed with the result that he persuaded Sir Robert Liston to carry out an amputation of a leg under

* Dr Gerald L Zeitlin, who has drawn attention to the erosion of the marble inscription on Morton's monument,[16] has informed us that the inscriptiion is situated on the four sides of the monument, the sequence when walking clockwise round the monument being 'Wm T.G. MORTON, Inventor and Revealer of Anesthetic Inhalation'. 'BEFORE WHOM In all time Surgery was Agony'. 'BY WHOM Pain in Surgery was averted and annulled. 'SINCE WHOM Science has control of Pain'. Subsequent research has shown that Fülop-Miller's imaginative description is far from the truth. Richard Patterson has provided evidence that Jackson's insanity was the result of cerebral damage and not drink.[17] Richard J Wolfe, in his detailed study of Morton's life (Tarnished Idol),[18] contends that Morton was a disreputable character who was solely interested in material gain, and that Jackson was not to blame for the controversy. But D Zuck, in a critical review of Tarnished Idol, shows that Wolfe's account is also biased.[19]

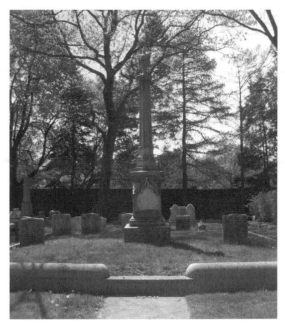

Figure 1.4 Morton's tombstone in Mount Auburn cemetery, Boston. (Reproduced with kind permission from a photograph taken by Dr Elliot V Miller MD, a retired senior staff member of the Massachusetts General Hospital Department of Anesthesia.)

ether anaesthesia. The operation was performed at University College Hospital, London on the 21 December 1846, the anaesthetic being given by a medical student, William Squire (Figures 1.6 and 1.7). Liston, who was known to be one of the fastest operators in London, took his usual 28 seconds to complete the job. It is interesting that one of the physicians at this hospital, John Elliotson, had been exploring 'mesmerism' and had suggested that it might be used to abolish the pain of surgery. However, he had been regarded as a quack and had been forced to resign his position. This explains Liston's comment after removing the leg: *'This Yankee dodge, Gentlemen, beats mesmerism hollow!'*.[20]

David Waldie, James Young Simpson and the switch from ether to chloroform in Great Britain

With the introduction of ether anaesthesia, James Young Simpson, Professor of Midwifery in Edinburgh, immediately seized on the

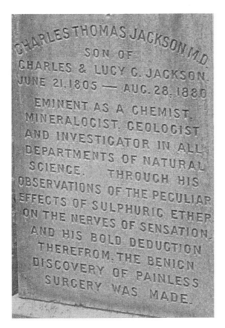

Figure 1.5 The inscription on Charles Jackson's tombstone. (Reproduced with the permission of the Department of Anesthesia, Massachusetts General Hospital.)

opportunity to use it for the relief of pain in childbirth. He began to use it within a few weeks of its first use for surgery in London, and, by doing so, ignited the religious and professional storm we discuss later (Chapter 20). Simpson became a champion for pain relief in labour, but he was not satisfied with ether and began a search for an agent that was more potent, less unpleasant to inhale and provided a more rapid induction. Simpson was friendly with another Edinburgh-trained doctor, David Waldie, who had prepared pure chloroform while working at the Society of Apothecaries in Liverpool. Waldie suggested that this might prove to be a suitable drug for Simpson to investigate.

Simpson and his colleagues had been sniffing a large number of substances in the hope that they would produce anaesthesia, and on 4 November 1847, he invited two of his assistants, James Matthews Duncan and George Keith, to dinner. Professor James Miller, a surgeon and friend, later described the scene. After the meal, they inhaled a number of volatile substances, one of which was chloroform. The drug

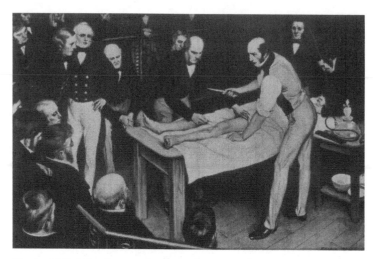

Figure 1.6 Painting by an unknown artist showing the first operation under ether anaesthesia at University College Hospital, London, 21 December 1846. (Reproduced with permission from University College London.)

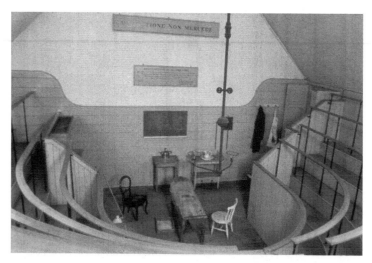

Figure 1.7 The operating theatre of the old St Thomas's Hospital, London, showing a wooden operating table from University College Hospital and the gallery for spectators. (Reproduced by kind permission of the Curator, The Old Operating Theatre, Museum and Herb Garret, London.)

proved to be very potent and the company became very loquacious before they became unconscious. When Simpson recovered consciousness:

> '... he turned round and saw Dr Duncan beneath a chair – his jaw dropped, his eyes staring, his head bent half under him, quite unconscious. And snoring in a most determined and alarming manner ... and then his eyes overtook Dr Keith's feet making valorous attempts to overturn the supper table, or more probably to annihilate everything that was on it'.[21]

One of the ladies present, Miss Petrie, Mrs Simpson's niece, then volunteered to inhale the vapour and began shouting *'I'm beginning to fly! I'm an angel! Oh, I'm an angel'*.[21]

On the next day, Simpson used the chloroform during labour, and five days later its successful use was reported to the Edinburgh Medical and Chirurgical Society. By 15 November, he had accumulated records of 50 cases in which he had used the drug. He lost no time in establishing his claim to fame. Indeed, he reserved for himself almost all of the credit for the discovery of chloroform anaesthesia, awarding Waldie a mere footnote in a later publication.[22]

Chloroform also had a pungent smell, but (unlike ether), it was non-explosive. It was also much more potent than ether, so induction of anaesthesia was much quicker. It was, however, very easy to give an overdose, and chloroform not infrequently produced irregularities of the heartbeat, and even cardiac arrest. Indeed, the first such death, in a 15-year-old girl, occurred within 11 weeks of the first use of the agent. A few patients also died from liver failure some days after the operation. Despite these risks, chloroform became a popular anaesthetic agent, particularly in Scotland. After John Snow, the first specialist anaesthetist, administered chloroform to Queen Victoria during the birth of Prince Leopold in 1853, it became fashionable to inhale small amounts during each contraction to reduce the pain of labour. Chloroform soon became a more popular agent than ether.[23] This continued to be the case in Scotland until the beginning of the 20th century, but in England the popularity of chloroform declined after the 1870s because of the high mortality rate associated with its use, and ether once again became the anaesthetic of choice. In the USA chloroform was rarely used, and ether reigned supreme (Figure 1.8). The last ether anaesthetic at the Massachusetts General Hospital was given on the 20 December 1979.*

---

* RJ Kitz, personal communication.

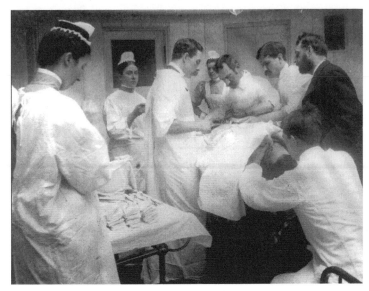

Figure 1.8 An operation in the Massachusetts General Hospital, Boston in 1908. The anesthetist (seated right) is dropping ether onto a facemask. This method was used for over a century. (Reproduced with the permission of the Department of Anesthesia, Massachusetts General Hospital.)

The further use of nitrous oxide

Although nitrous oxide was used for dental extractions in the 1840s, during the next 30 years most dental surgery was performed under chloroform or ether given by a nasal mask. The revival of interest in 'laughing gas' was brought about by Colton, the itinerant lecturer who had anaesthetized Wells for the extraction of his painful tooth. Colton formed the 'Colton Dental Association' in New York in the 1860s and subsequently set up branches in many other American cities. Colton later described how he had travelled to New Haven, Connecticut in 1863:

> *'... where, with the aid of Dr Smith* [a dentist] *we continued the business* [of extracting teeth] *for three weeks and two days, in which time we extracted something over three thousand teeth and stumps. This I thought was a little better business than lecturing, often to a "miserable account of empty boxes", and determined me to come to New York and establish an institution devoted exclusively to extracting teeth with the gas. As my name*

has been for so many years identified with laughing gas, I called it the "Colton Dental Association".

'It will be seen by the above that I claim no honour in the discovery of anaesthesia, that honour belongs to Dr Wells; but I confess to some pride in being the occasion of the discovery, and of having given the gas to Dr Wells for the first operation ever performed with an anaesthetic. If any honour is due to me, it is in reviving and establishing the use of the gas after it had lain dead and forgotten for twenty years'.[24]

In 1867, Colton travelled to Paris and reported that the gas had been given to some 24 000 patients without a death. His technique, which involved the inhalation of pure nitrous oxide from a bag, was learnt by TW Evans, a fashionable American dentist practising in Paris. Evans then travelled to London at his own expense and demonstrated the method at the Dental Hospital and several other places in London in March 1868. Since there was increasing concern about the safety of chloroform when given to patients in the dental chair at that time, the reintroduction of nitrous oxide proceeded apace.[25] Later in that year, cylinders containing the compressed and liquefied gas became available. In the same year, Edmund Andrews, a surgeon in Chicago, suggested that it should be given in combination with oxygen, but it was not until 1892 that the English anaesthetist Sir Frederick Hewitt introduced the first practical apparatus for administering the gas with oxygen.

The problem with nitrous oxide is that it a weak anaesthetic and may not produce unconsciousness unless given in such high concentrations that the supply of oxygen is severely restricted. The technique used for the three million or so dental anaesthetics given each year during the first half of the 20th century was to administer 95–100% nitrous oxide until the patient was unconscious, and then to cautiously increase the oxygen concentration to 8% or 10%. This technique invariably resulted in hypoxia. Since this could potentially damage the brain, many anaesthetists opposed the use of nitrous oxide in the dental chair, but it was not until the 1980s that the practice was finally abolished. Most of the dental surgery performed in the dental chair is now accomplished satisfactorily under local anaesthesia.

Afterword

Although some other inhalation agents were introduced in the late 19th and early 20th centuries, they proved to have disadvantages, and most patients continued to be anaesthetized with ether, chloroform or nitrous oxide up to the Second World War. Various inhalers were developed to facilitate the control of vapour concentration, but their use was restricted to some of the few specialist anaesthetists. In the UK, the majority of anaesthetics were given by a general practitioner, medical student or even the theatre porter; in contrast, in the USA, many anaesthetics were given by nurses under the instruction of the surgeon. The routine was to drop the volatile agent onto a gauze-covered mask placed over the mouth and nose. The induction was accompanied by a feeling of suffocation and dreaming, and patients had to be held down by several assistants while they passed through the stage of excitement and delirium into the stage of surgical anaesthesia. It was a most unpleasant experience, but one that the patient readily accepted in return for the blessed freedom from pain during surgery.

The discovery of general anaesthesia was one of the great medical advances of the 19th and 20th centuries. Six individuals deserve to share the credit, but only one is usually remembered. Disputes over priority were instrumental in the downfall or deaths of three: Wells, Morton and Jackson. Long, who had been the first to give surgical anaesthesia but had not reported it, failed in later efforts to claim priority and died a bitterly disappointed man. Colton and Simpson played important but secondary roles, and escaped relatively unscathed.

As Sir Frederick Treves commented in 1900, the introduction of general anaesthesia had a major effect on the development of surgery, but it was not until Lister's introduction of antisepsis in the mid-1860s and the subsequent adoption of aseptic techniques that mortality from surgery was drastically reduced. But, in 1884, there was another important advance in anaesthesia: the introduction of local anaesthesia with cocaine. Again there was controversy over priority, but it was much less destructive.

References

1. Hemlow J et al, eds. *The Journals and Letters of Fanny Burney (Madame d'Arblay)* Vol VI. *France 1803–1812*. Oxford: Clarendon Press, 1975: 596–616.
2. Ellis ES. *Ancient Anodynes*. London: Heinemann, 1946.
3. Cartwright FF. *The English Pioneers of Anaesthesia (Beddoes; Davy; Hickman)*. Bristol: Wright, 1952.
4. Bergman NA. Thomas Beddoes (1760–1808), tuberculosis and the medical pneumatic institution. In: Atkinson RS, Boulton TB, eds. *The History of Anaesthesia*. London: Royal Society of Medicine, 1989: 26–8.
5. Davy H. *Researches, Chemical and Philosophical: Chiefly Concerning Nitrous Oxide, or Dephlogisticated Nitrous Air, and its Respiration*. London: J Johnson, 1800.

6. Sykes WS. *Essays on the First 100 Years of Anaesthesia*. Vol 1. Edinburgh: Livingstone, 1960: 125.

7. Smith WDA. *Henry Hill Hickman*. UK: History of Anaesthesia Society, 2005.

8. Duncum BM. *The Development of Inhalation Anaesthesia: With Special Reference to the Years 1846–1900*. London: Oxford University Press, 1947: 77–89.

9. Ibid: 94–8.

10. Davison MHA. *The Evolution of Anaesthesia*. Altrincham: John Sherratt and Son, 1965: 127.

11. Keys TE. *The History of Surgical Anesthesia*. New York: Dover, 1963: 21–3.

12. Fülöp-Miller R. *Triumph Over Pain* (transl E and C Paul). New York: Bobbs-Merrill, 1938: 125.

13. Keys TE. *The History of Surgical Anesthesia*. New York: Dover, 1963: 25–7.

14. Clinic-of-the-month, conducted by Shapiro SL. The great ether controversy: a strange interlude in the history of American medicine. *The Eye, Ear, Nose and Throat Monthly* 1969;**48**:51–6.

15. Fülöp-Miller F. *Triumph over Pain* (transl E and C Paul). New York: Bobbs-Merrill, 1938: 320.

16. Zeitlin GL. Deterioration of the inscription on Morton's monument. *American Society of Anesthesiologists Newsletter* 2006;**70**:21–3.

17. Patterson R. Dr Charles Thomas Jacobson's aphasia. *Journal of Medical Biography* 1997;**5**:228–31.

18. Wolfe RJ. *Tarnished Idol: William Thomas Green Morton and the Introduction of Surgical Anesthesia*. Novato, CA: Norman Publishing, 2001.

19. Zuck D. *History of Anesthesia Society Proceedings* 2002;**30**:115–20.

20. Dawkins CJM. The first public operation carried out under an anaesthetic in Europe. *Anaesthesia* 1947;**2**:51–61.

21. Gordon HL. *Sir James Young Simpson and Chloroform (1811–1870)*. London: T Fisher Unwin, 1897.

22. Simpson JY. *Account of a new Anaesthetic Agent as a Substitute for Sulphuric Ether in Surgery and Midwifery. . . Communicated to the Medico-Chirurgical Society of Edinburgh at their meeting on 10th November 1847*. Edinburgh: Sutherland and Knox/London: Samuel Highley, 1847.

23. Stratmann L. *Chloroform: The Quest for Oblivion*. London: Sutton, 2003.

24. Duncum BM. *The Development of Inhalation Anaesthesia: With Special Reference to the Years 1846–1900*. London: Oxford University Press, 1947: 273–4.

25. Smith GB, Hirsch NP. Gardner Quincy Colton: pioneer of nitrous oxide anesthesia. *Anesthesia and Analgesia* 1991:**72**;382–91.

Further reading

Bowes JB. Mandrake in the history of anaesthesia. In: Atkinson RS, Boulton TB, eds. *The History of Anaesthesia*. London: Royal Society of Medicine, 1989: 477–81.

Bigelow HJ. Insensibility during surgical operations produced by inhalation. *Boston Medical and Surgical Journal* 1846;**35**:309–17.

Boot F. Surgical operations performed during insensibility produced by the inhalation of sulphuric ether. *Lancet* 1847;**i**:5–8.

Long CW. An account of the first use of sulphuric ether by inhalation as an anaesthetic in surgical operations. *Southern Medical and Surgical Journal. New Series* 1849;**5**:705–13.

Martin LVH. Another look at Dumfries. *Anaesthesia* 2004;**59**:180–7.

Smith WDA. *Under the Influence. A History of Nitrous Oxide and Oxygen Anaesthesia*. London: Macmillan, 1982.

Wynbrandt J. *The Excruciating History of Dentistry*. New York: St Martin's Press, 1998.

2 Local anaesthesia: Carl Koller, Sigmund Freud and cocaine

On 11 September 1884, a 27-year-old Viennese surgeon, Carl Koller, operated on a patient who had glaucoma, having anaesthetized the eye with an aqueous solution of cocaine. It was the first recorded administration of a local anaesthetic, and it opened up a new era in surgery. Others had noted the benumbing effects of ingested cocaine, and had even suggested its possible use in surgery, but it was Koller who demonstrated the feasibility of using this new type of anaesthesia.

The coca leaf

Cocaine is obtained from the bush *Erythroxylon coca*, which grows in Bolivia, Peru and Ecuador. For many centuries, the Indians have chewed the leaves in order to withstand strenuous working conditions, hunger or thirst. Available in Europe in leaf form since the mid-18th century, interest in the potential medicinal uses of cocaine dates from 1859 with the publication by Paolo Mantegazza of *Sulle virtu igienichee medicinali della coca,* a pamphlet extolling the plant as a 'great new remedy for disease'.[1] The active principle, an alkaloid, was isolated and became available the following year. The benumbing effects of chewing leaves of the coca plant were widely known – indeed they could hardly be missed. But no further attention was given until the Peruvian army surgeon Tomas Moreno y Mayz remarked in 1868 that the sensory paralysing effects of cocaine might be put to use in medicine. After experimenting with cocaine in frogs, he wrote: *'Can it be used as a local anesthetic? It is not possible to answer after so few experiments; the future will have to decide this'.*[2]

Twelve years later, Vassili von Anrep, a Russian nobleman and physician working at the Pharmacological Institute in Wurtzburg, reported his inability to feel a pinprick at the affected site after he injected cocaine into his arm subcutaneously. He also painted his tongue with a 1% solution of cocaine and noted the resultant loss of sensitivity, ending his report with the recommendation that cocaine should be used as a local anaesthetic. Four years later, in 1884, the suggestion was put to the test in a laboratory where Sigmund Freud, assisted by Carl Koller, both in their late 20s, were studying the neuropharmacology of cocaine.[2]

Freud versus Koller

Sigmund Freud, then 28 years old, seized on cocaine, which had just become available in purified form, as potential therapy in psychiatry. He had read of its use in treating morphine addiction, recommended in an obscure journal, the Detroit *Therapeutic Gazette*. Rushing into print, he claimed that *'cocaine was so powerful a specific to morphine-addiction as well as to alcoholism that inebriate asylums can be entirely dispensed with'*.[3] Freud also believed that cocaine would be useful in the treatment not only of psychiatric disease, but also of digestive disorders, typhoid fever, tuberculosis, syphilis and mercury poisoning.

Freud was aware of the numbing effects of ingested cocaine, and he instructed his friend Leopold Konigstein, an ophthalmologist, to *'investigate the question of how far the anaesthetizing properties of cocaine were applicable to diseases of the eye'*.[4] It does not appear that Freud had surgery in mind, and in any event Konigstein failed to follow it up. Whether Freud suggested to Koller the use of cocaine in surgery of the eye is in doubt. On the occasion of Koller's initial use on 11 September, Freud was on holiday with his fiancee, Martha Bernays. On his return, he wrote that *'Dr. Karl Koller, quite independently, happened upon* [his] *felicitous idea of inducing complete anesthesia of the cornea and conjunctiva by means of cocaine'*.[4] In later years, believing that credit for the discovery of local anaesthesia was rightly his, he blamed Martha, now his wife, for his absence on 11 September and bore a long-lasting grudge against her and against Konigstein in that Koller, not Freud, was now *'regarded as the discoverer of local anesthesia by cocaine'*.[4]

Koller gave a quite different account of his discovery. Writing later, he stated that in 1884:

> *'I was an intern and house surgeon on the staff of the Allgemeine Krankenhaus in Vienna. ... The immediate cause for my approaching the question of local anesthesia was the*

unsuitability of general anesthesia for eye operations; for not only is the cooperation of the patient greatly desirable ... but the sequelae of general narcosis – vomiting, retching and general restlessness ... frequently constitute grave danger to the operated eye. ...

'Sometime in the summer of 1884 Freud, who had become interested in the physiological systemic effects of cocaine, asked me to undertake with him a series of experiments. ... The fact that cocaine locally applied paralyzed the terminations and probably the fibres of the sensory nerves had been known for twenty-five years before it came to the attention of someone [Koller, himself] *interested and desirous of producing local anesthesia for the performance of operations. It is not correct, as was said at the time, that I discovered this important fact by accident, a drop of the solution coming by chance into my eye. ... When in the course of preparing for the physiologic experiments, I realized that I had in my possession the local anesthetic which I had been previously searching for, I went at once to* [the] *laboratory'.*[5]

What then happened was recounted some years later by a young laboratory assistant:

'One summer day in 1884, Dr Koller, at that time a very young man, was engaged in a piece of embryonic research. He stepped into Professor Stricker's laboratory, drew a small flask in which there was a trace of white powder from his pocket, and addressed me ... in approximately the following words: "I hope, indeed I expect, that this powder will anaesthetise the eye." "We'll find out about that right away," I replied. A few grains of the substance were thereupon dissolved in a small quantity of distilled water, a large, lively frog was selected from the aquarium and held immobile in a cloth, and now a drop of the solution was trickled into one of the protruding eyes. ... After about a minute came the great historic moment, I do not hesitate to designate it as such. The frog permitted his cornea to be touched and even injured without a trace of reflex action or attempt to protect himself – whereas the other eye responded with the usual reflex action to the slightest touch'.[2]

The operation and its sequelae

Following his experiments, Koller operated for glaucoma after placing cocaine on the surface of the eye. This was on 11 September 1884, four days before a meeting of ophthalmologists in Heidelberg. He immediately wrote a paper for presentation at the meeting. Unable to afford the trip to Heidelberg, his paper was presented by a friend and colleague, together with a demonstration of his experiments. News of Koller's paper was reported in America within weeks by Henry Noyes, who had attended the Heidelberg meeting. Writing in the New York *Medical Record*, Noyes predicted that '*The momentous value of the discovery seems likely to be in eye practice of more significance than has been the discovery of anesthesia by chloroform or ether in general surgery and medicine*'.[2]

William Halsted and the problem of addiction

The enormous potential for a wider use in surgery was recognized at once. Among the first to seize the opportunity were William Halsted, Richard Hall and their surgical colleagues at Roosevelt Hospital in New York. Halsted had been looking for a way to anaesthetize the skin, and had achieved some success with the subcutaneous injection of water. He and Hall quickly launched a series of brilliant experiments in which they demonstrated how, by injecting cocaine around a major sensory nerve, they could produce anaesthesia of the anatomical region supplied by that nerve. They immediately introduced this technique into their surgical practice, and thus, in 1885, became the first to demonstrate what subsequently became known as *regional anaesthesia*.[6]

With great success came great tragedy. In the best of medical tradition, Halsted and Hall had conducted their clinical experiments on themselves, and in the process had become addicted. Cocaine addiction had not been recognized at that time (Freud in Vienna, while experimenting widely with cocaine, initially refused to acknowledge the possibility of addiction; the American Surgeon General, William Alexander Hammond, was equally outspoken in his denial that cocaine is addictive).[7]

The introduction of a drug that could produce anaesthesia when injected offered an alternative to the dangers and undesirable side-effects of inhalation with ether or chloroform. Carl Ludwig Schleich, a Berlin surgeon, saw this as an opportunity to avoid general anaesthesia entirely. He demonstrated that it was possible to achieve satisfactory anaesthesia by infiltrating the tissues with large volumes of a very dilute cocaine solution, so minimizing the total dose and the risk of toxicity. Reporting his success at a meeting of surgeons in 1892, he denounced the use of general anaesthesia as morally and legally wrong. Instead of receiving the enthusiastic endorsement he anticipated, he was shouted off the podium and left in disgrace.[8] Nevertheless, and despite subsequent unpopularity, his advocacy of what came to be called *infiltration anaesthesia* led to its wide use. Over the next few years, surgeons started to inject cocaine to produce local anaesthesia at the site of the incision, but dosage was poorly controlled and toxic reactions (convulsions and cardiovascular collapse) were frequent.

Spinal and epidural anaesthesia

Since there was a delay before cocaine addiction was recognized, other doctors quickly began to explore the potential uses of cocaine. A New York neurologist, J Leonard Corning, was attracted to its potential use in the treatment of pain. Corning is believed to have visited Halsted's and Hall's laboratory and witnessed their experiments. In 1885, he reported that the injection of cocaine between the spines of two vertebrae in a dog resulted in broad, circumferential, bands of anaesthesia. It has been assumed that the cocaine was introduced through the dural sac into the cerebrospinal fluid. This would have represented the first spinal anaesthesia, and Corning himself did call it 'spinal anaesthesia'. Spinal puncture was not known at that time, however (it was achieved six years later by Heinrich Quincke), and subsequent study of Corning's notes indicates that the injection was outside the dural sac. Corning had inadvertently produced what appears to have been the first lumbar epidural anaesthesia. Corning, believing that he had demonstrated spinal anaesthesia, suggested that it might be used for pain relief during surgery, but no one took up his suggestion for another 13 years.[9]

It was in August 1898 that August Bier, a German surgeon who initiated the wearing of 'Tin Hats' in the German Army during the First World War, performed the first well-documented 'spinal anaesthesia'. Bier injected 3 ml of a 0.5% cocaine solution into the cerebrospinal fluid (CSF) of a patient to produce anaesthesia for a surgical operation. Over the next few days Bier and an assistant used the technique in a further six patients. To show their faith in the technique, they injected cocaine into each other's spinal fluid. As a result, Bier became the first to suffer a spinal headache due to the leakage of CSF through the hole in the dura made by a large-bore needle. Later, Bier abandoned the technique because of the toxicity of cocaine.

The search for a new drug

It soon became apparent that cocaine is not only highly toxic but also highly addictive. Cocaine had become widely available and was popular for its euphoria-producing effects. It was freely available over the counter at pharmacies and appeared in a wide variety of tonics, most notably Coca-Cola. By 1900, the public was in the throes of a cocaine epidemic. The urgent need for a local anaesthetic drug that was less toxic and non-addictive was taken up by a German research chemist, Alfred Einhorn. It took several years of painstaking research before he was able to synthesize a satisfactory substitute, a benzoic acid derivative that, combined with a basic alcohol, formed an organic salt that he called procaine.[10] Einhorn published his research in 1905, and later in the same year procaine was introduced clinically by Henreich Braun, a Leipzig surgeon. Procaine was immediately recognized as a much less toxic drug and, more importantly, it did not lead to addiction. It rapidly became widely used for spinal and other forms of local and regional anaesthesia. It was the forerunner of a number of longer-acting and still less toxic local anaesthetic drugs that have subsequently been introduced into clinical practice.

The use of local anaesthetic drugs lay entirely in the province of surgeons well into the 20th century. Whenever possible, surgeons conducted their own nerve blocks, not just to avoid the risks of general anaesthesia, but also to avoid the necessity of sharing responsibility with a physician– (or nurse–) anaesthetist. The Mayo Clinic in Rochester, Minnesota, played an important role in the recognition of the advantages of regional anaesthesia and ultimately in the transfer of responsibility to specialists in anaesthesia. In 1920, William Mayo recruited a young French surgeon, Gaston Labat, to introduce regional anaesthesia into his clinic. During his single year at the Mayo Clinic, Labat wrote what became the definitive textbook in America, *Regional Anesthesia: Its Techniques and Clinical Application*.[11] Following Labat's departure and a four-year interval under surgical administration, Mayo recruited a physician–anaesthetist to head the section on anaesthesia. The anaesthetist was John Lundy, who had had no experience in regional anaesthesia but who quickly learnt the techniques, and later established the foremost teaching and clinical programme in the USA.[12]

As recounted in later chapters, doctors specializing in anaesthesia replaced nurse–anaesthetists only slowly over the following years, and the transfer of the responsibility of local and regional anaesthesia from surgeons to anaesthetists was inevitably slow. As a result, surgeons continued to play the leading role in the development of new techniques. In 1921, Fidel Pagés Miravé, a Spanish surgeon, was the first to perform and describe the use of lumbar epidural anaesthesia for a surgical operation.[13] He died a year later in a traffic accident, and his priority remained unknown for many years. Ten years later in Italy, another surgeon, Achile Mario Dogliotti, unaware of Pagés's publication, described lumbar epidural anaesthesia, and for many years he was given the credit for its introduction.[14] Epidural anaesthesia has now largely replaced spinal anaesthesia for major abdominal surgery and is widely administered for control of pain in childbirth.

In recent years, the introduction of electrical nerve stimulators has increased the accuracy of nerve blocks, while improved needles and catheters and the addition of opiate drugs to the local anaesthetic have widened the scope of spinal and epidural anaesthesia. Since regional techniques avoid many of the complications associated with general anaesthesia and can provide significant pain relief into the postoperative period, there has been a great resurgence of interest in the use of local and regional anaesthesia in many branches of surgery. The patient who undergoes a cataract operation under regional anaesthesia in the morning and returns home in the afternoon has every reason to be grateful not only to Carl Koller, but also to that Viennese frog on which he first demonstrated the anaesthetic effects of that scourge of modern civilisation – cocaine.

References

1. Thornton EM. *Freud and Cocaine: The Freudian Fallacy.* London: Blond & Briggs, 1983.
2. Altman AJ, Albert DM, Fournier GA. Cocaine's use in ophthalmology: Our 100-year heritage. *Survey of Ophthalmology* 1985;**29**:300–6.
3. Musto DF. A study in cocaine: Sherlock Holmes and Sigmund Freud. *Journal of the American Medical Association* 1968;**204**:125–30.
4. Kuhn P. A professor through the looking-glass: contending narratives of Freud's relationship with the sisters Bernays. *International Journal of Psychoanalysis* 1999;**80**:943–59.
5. Koller C. Historical notes on the beginning of local anesthesia. *Journal of the American Medical Association* 1928;**90**:1742–3.
6. Halsted WS. Practical comments on the use and abuse of cocaine; suggested by its invariably successful employment in more than a thousand minor surgical operations. *New York Medical Journal* 1885;**42**:294–5.
7. Olch PD. William S Halsted and local anesthesia: contributions and complications. *Anesthesiology* 1975;**42**:479–86.
8. Goerig M. Carl Ludwig Schleich and the introduction of infiltration anesthesia into clinical practice. *Regional Anesthesia and Pain Medicine* 1998;**23**:538–9.
9. Cousins MJ, Bridenbaugh PO. *Neural Blockade in Clinical Anesthesia and Management of Pain.* Philadelphia: Lippincott-Raven, 1998.
10. Dunsky JL. Alfred Einhorn: the discoverer of procaine. *Journal of the Massachusetts Dental Society* 1997;**46**:25–6.
11. Labat G. *Regional Anesthesia: Its Techniques and Clinical Application.* Philadelphia, WB Saunders, 1922.

12. Pulido JN, Bacon DR, Rettke SR. Gaston Labat and John Lundy: friends and pioneer regional anesthesiologists sharing a Mayo Clinic connection. *Regional Anesthesia and Pain Medicine* 2004;**29**:489–93.
13. De Lange JJ, Cuesta Ma, Cuesta de Pedro A. Fidel Pagés Miravé (1886–1923): the pioneer of lumbar epidural anaesthesia. *Anaesthesia* 1994;**49**:429–43.
14. Dogliotti AM. Eine neue Methode der regionären Anäesthesie: die peridurale segmentäre Anästhesie. *Zentralblatt für Chirurgie* 1931;**58**:3141–5.

Further reading

Liljestrand G. Carl Koller and the development of local anaesthesia. *Acta Physiologica Scandinavica* 1967; **Suppl 299**: 1–30.

3 Entering the 20th century

For general anaesthesia to progress in the 20th century, it was necessary to develop an apparatus that could add ether or chloroform to a mixture of oxygen and nitrous oxide so that the concentration of volatile agent could be more accurately controlled. Second, it was necessary to devise a way in which an airtight connection could be made with the lungs so that the patient could receive the gas mixture undiluted with room air. Third, the anaesthetist had to learn how to maintain ventilation of the lungs when the patient's respiration became inadequate. And fourth, the anaesthetist had to devise a method of preventing collapse of the lungs when the surgeon wished to operate within the chest. It was the development of tracheal tubes in the 1920s that provided control of the airway, facilitated assisted and controlled ventilation, and opened the door for thoracic surgery, while control of ventilation was also facilitated by the development of carbon dioxide absorption breathing systems. Then, the introduction of intravenous anaesthesia with thiopental and, later, muscle relaxation with curare brought about a major revolution in anaesthetic practice. These changes are summarized in the time chart shown in Figure 3.1.

The anaesthesia machine

Although the pioneer anaesthetists such as Morton, Squire and Snow used specially designed vaporizers to deliver ether vapour to the patient, most anaesthetists administered ether and chloroform by dropping the liquid onto a gauze mask held over the face. Since there was no way of knowing what concentration of vapour was being inhaled, the anaesthetist learnt how to assess the depth of anaesthesia by observing changes in the pattern of respiration and the patient's response to surgery. It was Arthur Guedel, a remarkable American anaesthetist who used to visit forward surgical units on his motorcycle during the First World War,

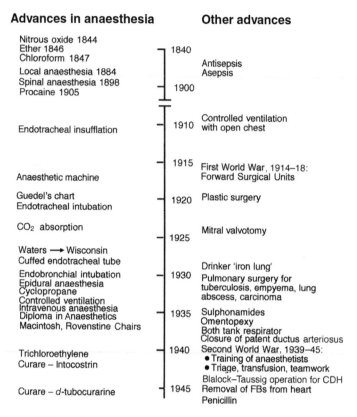

Advances in anaesthesia   **Other advances**

Advances in anaesthesia		Other advances
Nitrous oxide 1844		
Ether 1846	1840	
Chloroform 1847		Antisepsis
Local anaesthesia 1884		Asepsis
Spinal anaesthesia 1898	1900	
Procaine 1905		
		Controlled ventilation
Endotracheal insufflation	1910	with open chest
	1915	
		First World War, 1914–18:
Anaesthetic machine		Forward Surgical Units
Guedel's chart	1920	Plastic surgery
Endotracheal intubation		
CO$_2$ absorption		Mitral valvotomy
	1925	
Waters → Wisconsin		
Cuffed endotracheal tube		Drinker 'iron lung'
Endobronchial intubation	1930	Pulmonary surgery for
Epidural anaesthesia		tuberculosis, empyema, lung
Cyclopropane		abscess, carcinoma
Controlled ventilation		
Intravenous anaesthesia	1935	Sulphonamides
Diploma in Anaesthetics		Omentopexy
Macintosh, Rovenstine Chairs		Both tank respirator
		Closure of patent ductus arteriosus
Trichloroethylene	1940	Second World War, 1939–45:
Curare – Intocostrin		• Training of anaesthetists
		• Triage, transfusion, teamwork
		Blalock–Taussig operation for CDH
Curare – d-tubocurarine	1945	Removal of FBs from heart
		Penicillin

Figure 3.1 Time chart showing developments in anaesthesia and surgery from 1900–1945. CDH, congenital disease of the heart; FBs, foreign bodies.

who first produced a chart that illustrated how these signs changed with depth of anaesthesia and so enabled inexperienced doctors and medical orderlies to administer ether safely close to the front line (Figures 3.2 and 3.3).

The breathing of ether or chloroform vapour is very unpleasant, and, at the end of the 19th century, it was realized that anaesthesia could be induced more pleasantly and rapidly if the patient was put to sleep with nitrous oxide and oxygen, and the volatile agent then added to the gas mixture. The first machines designed to produce such a mixture were introduced by James Taylor Gwathmey in New York and by Geoffrey

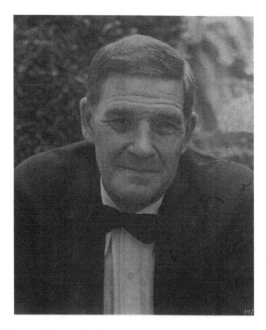

Figure 3.2 Arthur E Guedel (1883–1956) had to work his way through medical school, and despite losing three fingers from his right hand at the age of 13, became an accomplished pianist, organist and composer. He started to practise as a general practitioner–anaesthetist in 1909 and served in the American Expeditionary Force during the First World War. The medical services could not cope with the huge number of casualties, so Guedel trained nurses and orderlies to give simple, safe anaesthetics with ether, and frequently rode his motorbike to the forward units where they worked. (Reproduced with kind permission from The Wood Library–Museum of Anesthesiology, Park Ridge, Illinois.)

Marshall, who was serving in France in the First World War,[1] but it was the portable anaesthetic machine described in 1917 by Edmund Boyle, a Consultant Anaesthetist at St Bartholomew's Hospital in London, that became the forerunner of a sequence of Boyle's machines that were used until the late 1970s.[2] The compressed gases were stored in cylinders (Figure 3.4). Initially, there were no reducing valves to provide a constant gas pressure, so the flow decreased as the cylinder emptied and the anaesthetist had to continually readjust the flow control valves. Within a few years, reducing valves that maintained a constant output pressure,

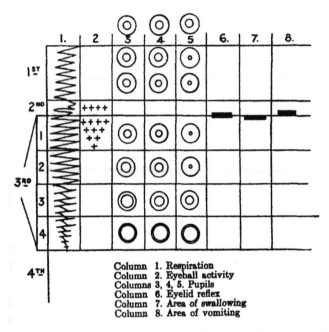

Column 1. Respiration
Column 2. Eyeball activity
Columns 3, 4, 5. Pupils
Column 6. Eyelid reflex
Column 7. Area of swallowing
Column 8. Area of vomiting

Figure 3.3 Chart provided by Guedel to help his trainees judge the depth of ether anaesthesia during the First World War. During the *first stage* (top), the patient is conscious but pain sensation is reduced. Probably some of the first operations under anaesthesia were performed in this stage. In the *second stage* (narrow band), the patient is unconscious but may be excited and uncontrollable. The onset of surgical anaesthesia in the *third stage* is marked by regular deep breathing. Superficial operations may be performed in *planes 1 and 2,* but anaesthesia must be deepened to *plane 3* to provide enough muscular relaxation for the surgeon to operate within the abdomen. As anaesthesia is deepened, the rib movements cease and breathing is maintained by the diaphragm so that abdominal movement persists until respiration ceases in the *fourth stage* (bottom). The pupils dilate and cease to react to light as anaesthesia is deepened. (Reproduced from Guedel AE. *Inhalation Anaesthesia. A Fundamental Guide.* New York: New Macmillan Co, 1945.)

and vaporizing bottles for ether and chloroform, were added to the machine. The vaporizers enabled the operator to increase the concentration of vapour gradually, thereby facilitating the induction of anaesthesia, but since there was no compensation for the cooling of the liquid as it evaporated, the anaesthetist still did not know what

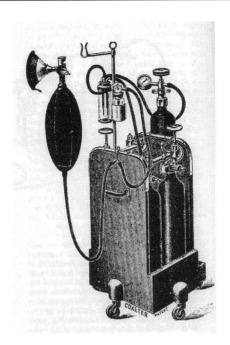

Figure 3.4 Boyle's anaesthetic machine (1917). The flow of oxygen and nitrous oxide from cylinders was controlled by needle valves attached to the cylinders and measured by two narrow metal tubes mounted vertically under water. Gas exited from each tube through a series of small holes, each of which transmitted 1 litre of gas per minute. Flow rate could be determined by counting the number of holes through which gas bubbled. The mixed gases were passed through an ether vaporizer to a reservoir bag, and expired gas escaped through a one-way valve close to the face mask. The nitrous oxide cylinder valve was heated by a spirit lamp to prevent freezing of the water vapour present in nitrous oxide as the gas expanded and cooled. (Reproduced with kind permission from the Association of Anaesthetists of Great Britain and Ireland from Watt OM. The evolution of the Boyle apparatus 1917–67. *Anaesthesia* 1968;**23**:103–18.)

concentration was being administered and had to judge the depth of anaesthesia on the basis of Guedel's signs. Temperature-compensated vaporizers that delivered a known concentration of the agent were not added to anaesthetic machines until the 1960s, when the potent non-explosive anaesthetic halothane (Fluothane) was introduced into clinical practice. The standard Boyle's machine of the 1930s (Figure 3.5) remained in use until the 1980s, when microprocessor-controlled

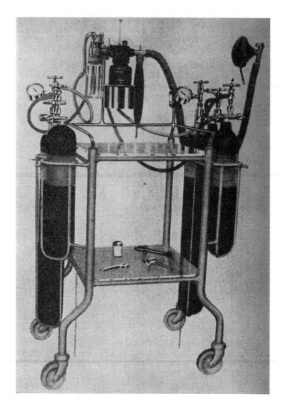

Figure 3.5 Standard Boyle machine used from the 1930s to the 1950s. It was fitted with a Magill breathing attachment with the reservoir bag on the machine. With an adequate fresh gas flow, carbon dioxide was eliminated through the expiratory valve. The anaesthetist could inflate the lungs by partially closing the spring-loaded expiratory valve and compressing the bag. (Reproduced with kind permission from the Association of Anaesthetists of Great Britain and Ireland from Watt OM. The evolution of the Boyle apparatus 1917–67. *Anaesthesia* 1968;**23**:103–18.)

machines with sophisticated monitoring of machine function were gradually introduced (see Chapter 18).

The airway during anaesthesia

When anaesthesia is induced, the tongue falls back and obstructs the airway. To avoid airway obstruction, the anaesthetist must tilt the head backwards and push the chin forwards throughout the period of unconsciousness; since the tongue is attached to the inside of the jaw, this pulls the tongue away from the back of the throat. If the nasal passages are blocked, it may also be necessary to insert a pharyngeal airway to maintain an opening through the mouth. Since a face mask prevents surgical access to the mouth, and it is difficult to hold a mask on the face and to push the chin forward for long periods, some other method of ensuring a clear airway had to be developed.

Although attempts had been made to pass a tube into the trachea for resuscitation purposes in the 18th century, it was not until 1880 that William MacEwen, Professor of Surgery in Glasgow, described how the fingers could be used to guide a tube into the larynx.[3] Then, in 1887, Joseph O'Dwyer, a children's specialist at the Foundling Hospital in New York, who had watched four of his sons die from diphtheria, described how he had inserted short, funnel-shaped tubes into the larynx to maintain a patent airway during the acute phase of the disease. O'Dwyer reported that out of the 50 patients with severe laryngeal obstruction that he treated with this technique, 12 recovered after periods of intubation lasting up to five days.[4] Franz Kuhn, an innovative head and neck surgeon working in Kassel, Germany, had probably heard of this work while visiting the USA, and, in the early 1900s, he wrote a series of papers advocating the use of a new flexo-metallic tube during anaesthesia. He realized that anaesthesia could be maintained at a lighter plane when a tube was in place, since the tube prevented reflex closure of the glottis in response to surgical stimuli. He was the first to describe the use of cocaine to provide topical anaesthesia of the larynx before intubation, and he was also the first to describe the use of a suction catheter to aspirate secretions from the trachea.[5] Since these papers were written in German, and not translated into English until the 1930s, it is Magill and Rowbotham who are generally credited with the introduction of tracheal intubation into anaesthesia.

Ivan Magill and Stanley Rowbotham

After the First World War, there were many ex-servicemen who had suffered horrific injuries to their face or jaw, so Harold Gillies, the founder of plastic surgery in Britain, set up a unit to perform reconstructive surgery in the Queen's Hospital for Facial and Jaw Injuries at Sidcup in Kent (Figure 3.6). In 1919, Ivan Magill and Stanley Rowbotham, two ex-army medical officers with little previous experience of anaesthesia, were appointed as anaesthetists to the unit (Figure 3.7). The injuries were diverse and the surgery involved multiple operations, so there were many problems for the anaesthetist.[6,7]

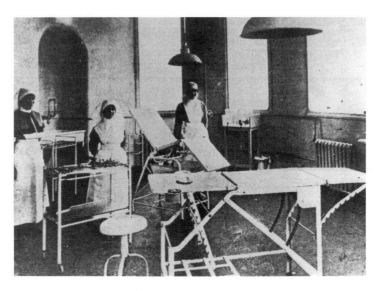

Figure 3.6 The operating theatre at the unit for facial injuries in Sidcup, Kent, in which Ivan Magill and Stanley Rowbottom administered anaesthesia to men wounded in the First World War. (Reproduced with kind permission from the Association of Anaesthetists of Great Britain and Ireland.)

In order to provide satisfactory operating conditions, Magill and Rowbotham were forced to develop new techniques for providing an airway and administering anaesthesia.[8] They started by using the insufflation technique, in which a high flow of nitrous oxide and oxygen with a volatile anaesthetic agent was blown down a narrow-bore tube into the trachea, and allowed to flow back out of the larynx.[9,10] Since the returning gas contained anaesthetic vapour and blew secretions and blood out through the mouth, the technique was not acceptable to the surgeon. Magill and Rowbotham then tried adding a wider return tube, but this also proved unsatisfactory. Finally, they decided to use a single large-bore tube. They fashioned these tubes from the standard rubber piping that was used to transport gas from the gas tap on the wall to the ubiquitous gas ring that heated the tea-kettle. The rubber pipe was stored in the form of a coil and so had a natural curve that made it easier to pass into the larynx.

Magill and Rowbotham developed two methods of inserting these tubes through the larynx into the trachea. The first technique was discovered by chance when a rather long curved tube, which had been inserted to maintain an airway through the nose, slipped into the trachea. Rowbotham found that if he added carbon dioxide to the anaesthetic gas

(a)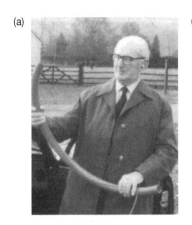

(b)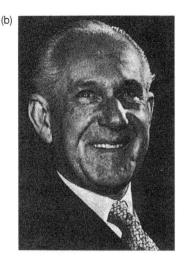

Figure 3.7 (a) Sir Ivan Magill with a tracheal tube designed for horses. (Reproduced with kind permission from a photograph taken by the late Dr JSM Zorab.) (b) Stanley Rowbotham, who described the technique of blind nasal intubation. (Reproduced with kind permission from the Association of Anaesthetists of Great Britain and Ireland from Condon HA, Gilchrist E. Stanley Rowbotham. Twentieth century pioneer anaesthetist. *Anaesthesia* 1986;**41**:46–52.)

mixture, he could stimulate respiration and so widen the larynx while he slipped the tube into the trachea.[11] This technique, known as blind intubation, proved to be of immense value, for it enabled the tube to be passed quickly under a light level of anaesthesia and, even more importantly, the trachea could be intubated when the vocal cords could not be visualized with a laryngoscope because of facial or neck deformity.

The second technique was to pass the tube under direct vision.[12] Magill developed a battery-powered laryngoscope and special forceps for this purpose (Figure 3.8a), but because this method was technically difficult and required deep anaesthesia to prevent reflex closure of the vocal cords, few anaesthetists attempted to pass a tube until the Second World War. Then, in 1943, Robert Macintosh, Professor of Anaesthetics at Oxford, and Richard Salt, Chief Technician (see Chapter 5), noticed that the surgeon had a good view of the larynx when a Boyle–Davis gag had been inserted to hold the mouth open during tonsil operations.[13] This gave them the idea of using a curved laryngoscope blade that lifted the base of the tongue instead of the epiglottis. This blade also gave them a better view of the vocal cords (Figure

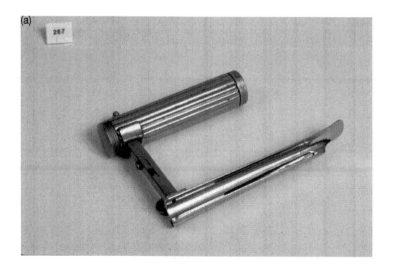

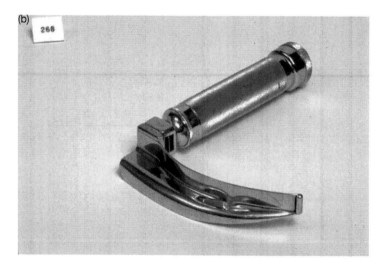

Figure 3.8 (a) Magill laryngoscope. The tip of the straight blade lifts the epiglottis, so enabling the anaesthetist to see the vocal cords. (b) Macintosh laryngoscope. The tip of the curved blade lifts the base of the tongue, and this tilts the epiglottis forward, so providing a good view of the vocal cords. Since the epiglottis is not touched, intubation can be performed under lighter anaesthesia. (Nuffield Department of Anaesthetics, Oxford).

3.8b). Since the base of the tongue is less sensitive than the epiglottis, intubation could be performed under lighter levels of anaesthesia. The Macintosh laryngoscope greatly facilitated intubation and helped to popularize the use of tracheal tubes during the later stages of the war.

Arthur Guedel and Ralph Waters

On the other side of the Atlantic, Arthur Guedel and Ralph Waters were also experimenting with tracheal tubes. Ralph Waters, of whom we shall hear much in later chapters, was the Head of the University Department of Anesthesia in Madison, Wisconsin, and had been friendly with Guedel for a number of years. Guedel (Figure 3.2) was the anaesthetist who had documented the signs of depth of anaesthesia to help the front-line medics in the First World War.

Although Guedel and Waters never lived in the same city, they met at meetings of the Anesthesia Travel Club and other societies, and corresponded regularly about their daily problems. Both were attempting to make a completely airtight breathing system so that Waters' carbon dioxide absorption breathing system (which had been introduced in 1924) could be used with a low flow of fresh gases, thus reducing the cost of each anaesthetic. Guedel experimented with rubber tubes fitted with inflatable balloons (now called cuffs) placed above, level with or below the vocal cords, and eventually decided to place the cuff on the part of the tube that lay in the trachea. Guedel and Waters published a description of this tube in 1928[14] and later proved its effectiveness by submerging his anaesthetized and intubated pet dog under water for an hour, and then allowing it to recover (Figure 3.9). On one of the occasions when this 'dunked dog' experiment was being demonstrated, a member of the audience recalled seeing another description of a tube with a cuff, so Waters and his colleagues performed a detailed literature search. This revealed that the idea of using an inflatable cuff was by no means new. They obviously found this kind of research to be very time-consuming, because they preface the report with the cryptic comment: '*The pleasure of this research has been exceeded only by the work involved*'.[15]

The laryngeal mask airway

In 1983, an English anaesthetist, Archibald Brain, introduced a device that revolutionised the maintenance of the airway during routine anaesthesia – the laryngeal mask airway.[16] This is a tube with a terminal cuff resembling a small facemask that can be inflated to provide an airtight seal around the entrance to the larynx. The airway can be inserted into the pharynx without using a laryngoscope under light anaesthesia and is now used routinely in patients when there is no specific indication for tracheal intubation. It is relatively easy to insert, avoids damage to the larynx, and has proved lifesaving in the emergency situation and when tracheal intubation is difficult.

Anaesthesia for thoracic surgery

With compressed gases from the anaesthetic machine and cuffed tracheal tubes to provide an airtight connection with the lungs, anaesthetists could now ventilate the lungs by compressing the reservoir bag in the breathing system. But, even more importantly, they could deal with the problem posed by the open chest. When the surgeon opens the chest, the elasticity of the lungs causes them to collapse and air rushes in to fill the pleural space between the lungs and chest wall. The alveolae empty within minutes and the uptake of oxygen and elimination of carbon dioxide cease. Whereas the inflated lung looks like a pink sponge, the collapsed lung looks like a piece of liver. To keep the patient alive, the anaesthetist must prevent lung collapse and also maintain the normal ventilation of the lungs so that oxygen and carbon dioxide are exchanged normally.

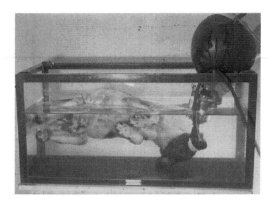

Figure 3.9 Photograph of 'dunked dog' experiment originally performed by Arthur Guedel. The dog used in this demonstration to students was called 'Airway' and had been given to Waters' two sons as a present. It was anaesthetized with ether and intubated with a cuffed tube that provided an airtight seal with the trachea. The tube was then connected to a Waters carbon dioxide absorption canister (right, at water level) and anaesthetic machine. The dog remained under water throughout the demonstration, and showed no after effects on recovering consciousness. (Reproduced with kind permission from the Wood Library–Museum of Anesthesiology, Park Ridge, Illinois.)

There were many attempts to overcome the problem posed by the open chest. The most expensive – and the most ineffectual – approach to the problem was that pioneered by the young German surgeon Ferdinand Sauerbruch of Breslau,[16] who was assistant to the great surgeon von Mikulicz. He enclosed both patient and surgeon in an operating room in which the air pressure was maintained at a level that was less than atmospheric, while the patient's head and the anaesthetist were outside the chamber. When the chest was opened, the constant pressure difference between the inside and outside of the lung maintained lung expansion, but since there was no cyclical variation in pressure, ventilation was entirely dependent on the movement of the lung on the unopened side. Because of mediastinal shift, the chest wall movements produced little ventilation, so the level of carbon dioxide in the blood increased, thus limiting the duration of anaesthesia. Later, anaesthetists recognized that the high gas flow used in the insufflation technique introduced by Melzer and Auer[9,10] kept the lungs inflated by creating a positive pressure in the trachea, but again the constant pressure provided no assistance to ventilation. Although some ventilation could be provided by periodically interrupting the gas flow, and allowing the lung to partially deflate, the method fell into disuse.

It was Janeway and Green in the USA who demonstrated in animals that the application of *intermittent* positive pressure to the trachea could produce enough ventilation to maintain carbon dioxide homeostasis without interference with the circulation.[18] Furthermore, lung collapse could be prevented by maintaining a small residual positive pressure during expiration.*

It was this technique that anaesthetists began to adopt in the 1920s. Initially they 'assisted ventilation' by compressing the reservoir bag on the anaesthetic machine in time with the patient's inspiration: by adjusting the residual pressure in the bag during expiration, they could maintain the appropriate degree of lung expansion. This technique enabled normal oxygen and carbon dioxide levels to be maintained throughout long operations. Later, as Janeway and Green had discovered, anaesthetists found that if they lowered the carbon dioxide level by a period of increased ventilation, the patient's spontaneous breathing could be arrested. This enabled the anaesthetist to hold the lung motionless while the surgeon performed some delicate manoeuvre. The technique of 'controlled ventilation' in which the patient's lungs are ventilated

---

* Although the work of Janeway and Green made thoracic surgery possible, neither continued to work in this field: Janeway became a general surgeon and Green became a radiologist.

rhythmically in the absence of any spontaneous breathing is now routine, and will be referred to frequently in ensuing chapters.*

There was one other important advance: the development of carbon dioxide absorption breathing systems. Waters introduced his to-and-fro absorption system in 1924 and Brian Sword described the circle system in 1930. Since these eliminated the need for a high flow of fresh gas to flush the expired carbon dioxide out of the system, fresh gas flow could be reduced, thereby decreasing the costs of an anaesthetic. The use of such a system became essential when the highly explosive and expensive anaesthetic gas cyclopropane was introduced in 1934. With potent anaesthetics such as ether and cyclopropane, the breathing system could be completely closed and the fresh gas flow reduced to the basal oxygen requirement of about 300 ml/min.

So, by the beginning of the Second World War, the few anaesthetists who specialized in anaesthesia had learnt how to intubate the trachea and to control ventilation, although they had no means of assessing whether or not ventilation was adequate. They had two potent explosive anaesthetics – ether and the recently introduced gas cyclopropane – and two non-explosive agents – the weak nitrous oxide and the potent chloroform. But they were also beginning to use the drug that anaesthetists had been seeking for over a quarter of a century. That drug was thiopental, better known by its proprietary name, Pentothal. This brought about the first major revolution in anaesthetic practice in the 20th century.

Intravenous anaesthesia

Although it might take 30 minutes or more to induce anaesthesia with open-drop ether, inhalation anaesthesia did have the advantage that the concentration of the anaesthetic agent in the blood, which determines the depth of anaesthesia, could be controlled by varying the inspired concentration. The level of anaesthesia could therefore be varied to match the surgical requirements: light anaesthesia for superficial operations and deep anaesthesia when the surgeon required muscular relaxation to enable him to operate within the abdomen. Furthermore, when the administration was stopped, the blood concentration decreased and the patient recovered consciousness. Thus, uptake and elimination were under the control of the anaesthetist. In contrast, the injection of an

---

* Waters actually called this 'controlled respiration', but we now use the term 'ventilation' to describe the movement of gas in and out of the lungs. The term 'respiration' is used to describe all of the processes involved in the exchange of gases between the atmosphere and the body cells.

anaesthetic drug into a vein results in a rapid and unpredictable rise in the blood concentration, and the drug then remains in the body until it is either broken down by the liver or excreted through the kidneys. The rapid rise in blood concentration can result in dramatic changes in the patient's condition (for example, cessation of breathing or a profound fall in blood pressure), and the delayed excretion of the drug or its breakdown products can lead to a prolonged recovery.

The first experiments on the intravenous injection of drugs were carried out in the 17th century. William Harvey published his classic work *De motu cordis* ('On the Motion of the Heart') in 1628, but his conclusion that the blood circulates round the body and does not pulse in and out of the heart, as was previously believed, was a source of controversy for many years. Some 30 years later, Robert Boyle, John Wilkins and Christopher Wren, three of the founders of the Royal Society, were discussing the implications of this concept in relation to their interest in poisoning. They realized that if the poison from a scorpion's sting or a viper's bite were to enter the bloodstream, it would circulate round the body in seconds. Wren thought that he could test this hypothesis by injecting substances directly into a vein. He used a pig's bladder connected to a quill to inject a warm solution of white wine and opium into the vein in the hind leg of a dog. In an undated letter (*c*.1656–58) to his friend William Petty, he wrote:

> '... *I have injected Wine and Ale in a living Dog into the Mass of Blood by a Veine, in good Quantities, till I have made him extremely drunk, but soon after he pissith it out: with 2 ounces of infusion of Crocus Metall* [*Crocus mettalorum*, an emetic]*: thus injected, the Dog immediately fell a vomitting, and so vomited till he died. It will be too long to tell you the effects of Opium, Scammony, & other things I have tried in this way: I am now in further pursuit of the Experiment, which I take to be of great concernment, and what will give great light both to the Theory and Practice of Physick'.*[19]

He was right about the impact of the experiment on medicine, and reported it to the Royal Society in 1665. It was then argued that if harmful substances could be injected into the bloodstream, it should also be possible to inject substances that improved the blood. These arguments led to Richard Lower's experiments on blood transfusion in 1666, and ultimately to intravenous anaesthesia.

In the late 19th and early 20th century, a number of hypnotic drugs were being injected intravenously in attempts to produce sleep, and by the 1930s anaesthetists working in the London private clinics were administering barbiturate drugs such as pentobarbital (proprietary name Nembutal) to achieve a deep sleep so that the patient did not remember the horrors of an induction with gas, oxygen and ether. Since such drugs were long-acting and had other undesirable side-effects, the practice was not common elsewhere. Then, in 1932, Helmutt Weese, a clinical pharmacologist in Dusseldorf, Germany, introduced the first effective short-acting intravenous drug, hexobarbital (Evipan). This was quickly followed by the introduction of an even shorter-acting drug, thiopentone – now called thiopental (Pentothal). Thiopental soon became the standard drug used for induction of anaesthesia, and continued to be the most popular intravenous agent until the end of the 20th century.

Within a few years the hazards of intravenous anaesthesia were dramatically publicized. On the 7 December 1941, some 200 Japanese aircraft attacked the American Fleet anchored in Pearl Harbor. The USA suffered over 3400 casualties, with 2300 deaths. Most of the medical staff had no experience of war, and little knowledge of anaesthesia, but they were forced to provide anaesthesia for emergency surgery under very difficult circumstances, so most of the doctors chose to use thiopental as the sole anaesthetic agent. Since thiopental is a hypnotic and not a general anaesthetic, it was necessary to administer large doses to keep the patient immobile during the operation. Many of the patients had lost blood and were already in a state of surgical shock, and there were a number of deaths attributed to the anaesthetic.[20] Thiopental was then a relatively new drug, and it was not appreciated that the dose needed to establish unconsciousness was much lower in shocked patients. It now appears that the number of deaths caused by thiopental at Pearl Harbor was over-estimated, but the experience taught anaesthetists that thiopental should only be used as an induction agent, and then only in small doses.[21] Since that time, thiopental has been used successfully in many disaster situations where it would have been impossible to give an inhalation anaesthetic.[22]

The intravenous induction agents completely altered the patient's experience of anaesthesia, for they induced a pleasant sleep within a few seconds of the injection. If an appropriate dose was given, the patient recovered consciousness rapidly on completion of surgery and postoperative vomiting was greatly reduced. But these drugs were only designed to produce sleep, and did not provide any pain relief. To maintain unconsciousness and pain relief throughout the operation, they had to be followed by nitrous oxide and oxygen supplemented by narcotic drugs or by a volatile anaesthetic agent.

There was one other requirement for the successful use of intravenous anaesthesia, namely the development of a device that could be left in the vein for long periods without damaging the vein wall. Initially, the needle was surrounded by a thin metal cannula. The needle and cannula were threaded into the vein and the needle then withdrawn, leaving the blunt-ended cannula within the vein. This system was used from the 1940s until the 1960s, and greatly facilitated the administration of fluid and blood. The development of a similar system but with a thin plastic outer cannula is attributed to anesthesiologists at the Mayo Clinic in the mid-1950s, but it was not until the early 1960s that manufacturing problems were overcome and the use of this type of device became routine. Subsequently, improvements in materials and manufacturing techniques led to the development of an astonishing variety of plastic cannulae that are now used in all branches of medical practice.[23]

Curare and 'balanced anaesthesia'

As we shall learn in Chapters 8–10, the introduction of the muscle relaxant drug curare into anaesthetic practice in 1942 was one of the most important events in the history of anaesthesia. The use of curare enabled the three components of general anaesthesia – unconsciousness, pain relief and muscular relaxation – to be provided by separate drugs: unconsciousness was induced by thiopental and maintained by nitrous oxide; pain relief was provided by nitrous oxide supplemented by an intravenous analgesic drug such as morphine or pethidine, or a small concentration of a volatile agent; and muscular relaxation was induced by curare or some other muscle-relaxant drug. The advantage of this concept of so-called 'balanced anaesthesia' is that it enables the anaesthetist to adjust the dosage of each drug to provide the most appropriate conditions for the type of surgery being performed. Since the prolonged inhalation induction is avoided, the surgeon can operate within a few minutes of the intravenous injection, and, since the dose of each drug is minimized, side-effects are reduced, recovery hastened, and the incidence of postoperative complications reduced.

The new technique of thiopental, curare, tracheal tube, nitrous oxide–oxygen and an intravenous analgesic drug necessitated a high degree of technical skill and a much greater understanding of physiology and pharmacology than had been required for the administration of ether. Those who mastered the new knowledge found that they were in complete control of the patient and capable of coping with the expanding horizons of the surgical specialities. Surgeons were quick to realize the potential of the new technique and were able to undertake more invasive operations in much sicker patients.

The transition from the prolonged induction and heaving, tight abdomen associated with an ether anaesthetic to the rapid onset of unconsciousness and muscle relaxation provided by an intravenous induction with thiopental and curare was an important factor in creating the new relationship between the surgeon and the anaesthetist that developed after the Second World War. It was soon recognized that such anaesthetics could only be given safely by those who were properly trained, and this provided a further stimulus for the development of higher academic standards in the post-war period.

Before the first century of anaesthesia closed, however, there were two other developments that had a major influence on the subsequent development of the speciality. The first was the creation of an academic base for the subject, and the second was the influence of the Second World War.

References

1. Restall J. Military anaesthesia and the transport of casualties. In: Atkinson RS, Boulton TB, eds. *The History of Anaesthesia*. London: Royal Society of Medicine, 1989: 192–5.
2. Watt OM. The evolution of the Boyle apparatus. 1917–67. *Anaesthesia* 1968;**23**:103–18.
3. MacEwen W. Clinical observations on the introduction of tracheal tubes by the mouth instead of performing tracheotomy or laryngotomy. *British Medical Journal* 1880;**ii**:122–4,163–5.
4. O'Dwyer J. Fifty cases of croup in private practice treated by intubation of the larynx, with a description of the method and of the dangers incident thereto. *The Medical Record* 1887;**32**:557–61.
5. Kuhn F. *Die perorale Intubation*. Berlin: Verlag von S Karger, 1911.
6. Pallister WK. Sir Ivan Whiteside Magill (1888–1986) and tracheal intubation. In: Atkinson RS, Boulton TB, eds. *The History of Anaesthesia*. London: Royal Society of Medicine, 1989: 605–9.
7. Condon HA, Gilchrist E. Stanley Rowbotham. Twentieth century pioneer anaesthetist. *Anaesthesia* 1986;**41**:46–52.
8. Rowbottom S, Magill I. Anaesthetics in the plastic surgery of the face and jaws. *Proceedings of the Royal Society of Medicine* 1921;**14**:17–27.
9. Meltzer SJ, Auer JL. Continuous respiration without respiratory movements. *Journal of Experimental Medicine* 1909;**11**:622–5.
10. Kelly RE. Anaesthesia by the intratracheal insufflation of ether. *British Medical Journal* 1912;**ii**:112–14.
11. Rowbotham S. Intratracheal anaesthesia by the nasal route for operations on the mouth and lips. *British Medical Journal* 1920;**ii**:590–1.
12. Magill I. Endotracheal anaesthesia. *Proceedings of the Royal Society of Medicine* 1928;**22**:83–8.
13. Macintosh RR. A new laryngoscope. *Lancet* 1943;**i**:485.
14. Guedel AE, Waters RM. A new intratracheal catheter. *Current Researches in Anesthesia and Analgesia* 1928;**7**:238–9.
15. Waters RM, Rovenstine EA, Guedel AE. Endotracheal anaesthesia and its

historical development. *Current Researches in Anesthesia and Analgesia* 1933;**12**:196–203.

16. Brain AI. The laryngeal mask – a new concept of airway management. *British Journal of Anaesthesia* 1983;**55**:801–5.

17. Sauerbruch F. *Master Surgeon*. New York: Crowell, 1954.

18. Janeway HH, Green NW. Experimental intrathoracic esophageal surgery. *Journal of the American Medical Association* 1909;**53**:1975–8.

19. Tinniswood A. *His Invention So Fertile. A Life of Christopher Wren*. London: Jonathan Cape, 2001: 36.

20. Halford FJ. A critique of intravenous anesthesia in war surgery. *Anesthesiology* 1943;**4**:67–9.

21. Bennetts FE. Thiopentone anaesthesia at Pearl Harbour. *British Journal of Anaesthesia* 1995;**75**:366–8.

22. Dundee JW, Wyant GM. *Intravenous Anaesthesia*, 2nd edn. London: Churchill Livingstone, 1988.

23. Rivera AM, Strauss KW, van Zundert A, Mortier E. The history of peripheral intravenous catheters: how little plastic tubes revolutionized medicine. *Acta Anaesthesiologica Belgica* 2005;**56**:271–82.

Further reading

Benumof JL. *Anesthesia for Thoracic Surgery*. London: WB Saunders, 1987:1–14.

Bodman R. Cyclopropane and the development of controlled ventilation. In: Atkinson RS, Boulton TB, eds. *The History of Anaesthesia*. London: Royal Society of Medicine, 1989: 216–21.

Gillespie N. *Endotracheal Anesthesia*, 3rd edn. Madison: University of Wisconsin Press, 1963.

Mushin WW, Rendell-Baker L. *The Principles of Thoracic Anaesthesia*. Oxford: Blackwell Scientific, 1953.

Part 2

Professionalism in anaesthesia: the reluctant universities and the Second World War

In the period up to the Second World War, most of the anaesthetics in the UK were given by general practitioner–anaesthetists, junior hospital doctors, or medical students. The general practitioner–anaesthetists, surgeons and physicians received no fee for their work in the voluntary hospitals but hoped that the status of a hospital appointment would result in fees from private practice. Since the surgeon usually billed the patient, the anaesthetist was at his mercy and was lucky to receive 5% of the surgical fee. Anaesthetists therefore relied on general practice to supply most of their income.

The situation in the USA was different, because many surgeons employed nurses to administer the anaesthetics. The full-time nurse–anaesthetists were often more skilful than a doctor who only gave anaesthetics infrequently, they were cheaper, and they did not argue with the surgeon. Since private fees were relatively low, there was little incentive for a doctor to become an anaesthetist.

There were two major developments that completely changed the status of the anaesthetist between the 1930s and the postwar period. These were the development of an academic base for the subject and the experience gained in the Second World War. They set the scene for the widespread adoption of the thiopental–nitrous oxide–curare sequence already described. First we look at the way in which universities in the USA and the UK responded to the idea of an academic department of anaesthesia.

4 Ralph Waters pursues a vision (and succeeds)

Ralph Waters was the head of the first university department of anaesthesia (founded in 1927), and became a full professor in 1933. Robert Macintosh was the first professor appointed to an endowed chair in anaesthesia (1937). But long before either of these appointments, another physician, Henry Isaiah Dorr, had already begun to implement a vision of a scientific university-based study of anaesthesia. Dorr, a veteran of the American Civil War, believed in science as a force to advance social welfare. Coupled with a reverence for science was a profound compassion stemming from the suffering he had encountered in the war. In 1910, he offered Harvard University the income from an endowment of $63 000 to establish 'a Henry Isaiah Dorr Chair of Research and Teaching in Anaesthetics and Anaesthesia for the benefit of the Medical and Dental students of Harvard College and suffering humanity'. The bequest, initially rejected, was accepted when a larger endowment was offered. In 1927, the Chair was established, but the medical school had little interest in a chair in anaesthesia. It remained vacant until 1941, when Henry Knowles Beecher became the first Dorr Professor. The specific contributions of Waters and Beecher to the practice of anaesthesia are discussed in other chapters. Here we consider their role in the development of anaesthesia as an academic subject.

In the early part of the 20th century, there were only a few doctors in the USA who devoted all or most of their professional energies to anaesthesia. Many of these men and women had drifted from general practice into this new specialty as a way to supplement their incomes. Some clearly were attracted to what anaesthesia had to offer, while others were simply attempting to escape from the responsibilities of an unsuccessful or bothersome practice. But there were also a few who saw the opportunity to develop a new medical discipline. Their leader and spokesman was an articulate, dedicated and fiery doctor named Francis Hoeffer McMechan (Figure 4.1), and among his followers were Arthur Guedel and Ralph Waters.[1]

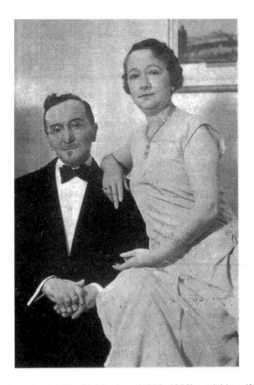

Figure 4.1 Francis Hoeffer McMechan (1879–1939) and his wife Laurette. McMechan was a very dedicated anaesthetist whose career was terminated by the early onset of severe rheumatoid arthritis that confined him to a wheelchair. Despite the severe physical constraints imposed by the worsening disease, McMechan, ably supported by his indomitable wife, continued his self-appointed task of improving the status of anaesthesia. He founded the National (later, International) Anesthesia Research Society and edited its journal *Current Researches in Anesthesia and Analgesia* from 1922 until his death in 1939. He organized conferences, continually opposed the employment of nurse–anesthetists, and worked tirelessly to further all aspects of academic anaesthesia.[1] (Reproduced with kind permission from Wood Library–Museum of Anesthesiology, Park Ridge, Illinois.)

Ralph Milton Waters

The practice of anaesthesia was built on its techniques. It was their skill in administering an ether anaesthetic or passing a tracheal tube that established the clinical reputations of Ralph Waters, the first Professor of Anesthesia at the University of Wisconsin, and Robert Macintosh, the first Nuffield Professor of Anaesthetics at the University of Oxford. The French surgeon Gaston Labat brought the techniques of regional anaesthesia to the Mayo Clinic in 1920, paving the way for the renowned school of regional anaesthesia subsequently developed by John Lundy.[2] The strength of the new discipline clearly lay in its techniques, but this was also a source of weakness. The importance of technical aspects in the practice of anaesthesia had been emphasized to the exclusion of intellectual and scientific components. In the inevitable comparison with medicine and surgery, the techniques of anaesthesia seemed meagre indeed.

Ralph Waters was the first to see beyond the technical limits of anaesthesia and to recognize and articulate the need for a scientific approach to the solution of problems he encountered in its clinical administration.[1] Research in anaesthesia at that time was carried out largely by pharmacologists in the laboratories of university medical schools. Waters clearly recognized that the development of the science and practice of anaesthesia must be brought to the university, so he set out to find one. His search resulted in the famous programme he built at the University of Wisconsin.

Waters arrived at the University in February 1927, and from that time until his retirement in 1948, Madison was a mecca for physician–anaesthetists. From Waters's programme sprang a generation of academic leaders. The Waters vision of academic anaesthesia probably reached its fullest expression in the Nuffield Department of Anaesthetics at Oxford that Robert Macintosh patterned closely on the programme at Madison, but there were many others who were inspired by the Waters ethos and patterned their departments on his ideals.

Macintosh and Waters were remarkably similar in medical background and personality. Both were skilful and shrewdly practical clinicians who brought the best of the practice of anaesthesia of their day to the university. Didactic teaching and research were added later. Henry K Beecher, the first Dorr Professor of Research in Anaesthesia at Harvard University, took an opposite approach. He began with research, picking up the practice of anaesthesia along the way. Although the goals were the same, the routes chosen were sufficiently different that the programme at Harvard was developed almost completely in isolation from those in Wisconsin and Oxford. Yet it was Beecher, among these 'first-generation' academic giants, who came closest to achieving the Waters goal of the application of the scientific method to the clinical practice of anaesthesia.

Waters had the vision, Macintosh adopted it on a glorious scale, and Beecher refined it to a level of high academic achievement. They could not, of course, do this single-handedly. A large measure of their success derived from the prestige of the distinguished universities they represented. Yet, however proud Wisconsin, Oxford and Harvard may be today of the brilliant achievements of these men, it is curious to note that of the three, only the University of Wisconsin had any interest in anaesthesia at the outset.

As a young doctor in Sioux City, Iowa, in 1913, Ralph Waters was one of about a hundred general practitioners. It was common to engage in some specialty work on the side, and Waters attempted to combine obstetrics and anaesthesia. When he realized that it was not possible to practise both specialities simultaneously, he chose to limit himself to anaesthesia. To encourage business, Waters rented a suite in a medical office building and opened a commercial venture that he called 'The Downtown Anesthesia Clinic'. A small operating room contained dental and surgical equipment and a sterilizer. Surgeons and dentists were invited to bring their patients to the clinic, in which complete operating room facilities were provided, including, of course, anaesthesia for the patient.

In 1923, Waters accepted an invitation to move to Kansas City, Missouri, where the use of physician–anaesthetists was already well established. An additional attraction was the prospect of proximity to the University of Kansas. Waters had already set his sights on a university-based anaesthesia programme, and by 1926 he was in the process of exploring the potential at the university when he seriously injured his back 'lifting a patient who weighed 325 pounds'.

Faced with six months of incapacity in a brace, Waters decided to visit John Lundy, who had already established the Anesthesia Section at the Mayo Clinic in Rochester, Minnesota (see below), to learn some of the regional block techniques for which the Clinic was already famous. Returning home from Rochester in late 1926, he stopped in Madison to visit his sister and her husband, Professor Erwin G Hastings of the Wisconsin School of Agriculture.

Through the Hastings, Waters met Joseph Evans, their personal physician and Professor of Medicine at the newly opened medical school. Waters already knew something of the new medical school from Chauncey Leake, a young pharmacologist there who was investigating the clinical effects of diethyl ether and who rubbed shoulders with practising anesthesiologists at medical meetings. Waters jumped at the opportunity to question Professor Evans about the possibility of an anaesthesia programme. The situation seemed almost ideal to Waters. He was particularly eager to develop a programme of pharmacological and physiological research and to collaborate with the distinguished basic science faculty at the medical school. Dean Charles Bardeen had known one of the early anesthesiologists, John J Buettner, in Syracuse, New York, and was favourably disposed to the new specialty, and in Erwin Schmidt, Professor of Surgery, Waters found an immediate ally. Schmidt was having difficulties with his nurse–anesthetists and was only too glad to have the bright young anesthesiologist undertake to solve the problem.

On 9 December 1926, Dean Bardeen wrote to Glenn Frank, president of the university, recommending Waters's appointment and commenting that '*we believe that this appointment will enable the university to make a real advance in an important field at present greatly neglected in the medical schools of the country*'.

On 20 January 1927, Ralph Waters was appointed Assistant Professor of Anesthesia at a salary of $4500 a year. The appointment notice read, in part, that he had '*devoted himself for a number of years to anesthetics as a Specialist at Kansas, Missouri. This is one of the few cities in the country in which the giving of anesthetics is accepted as a medical specialty rather than a specialty for nurses. He is recognized as foremost in his field*'. On 1 February, Waters reported for duty at the Wisconsin State Hospital (Figure 4.2).

Waters made many fundamental advances in anaesthetic practice. He advocated the use of carbon dioxide absorption techniques so that economies could be made by using smaller fresh gas flows, and later he found that the absorption of carbon dioxide enabled ventilation to be controlled, so improving operating conditions for the surgeon. He reintroduced the cuffed tracheal tube, and was the first to use endobronchial intubation so that one lung could be ventilated independently during thoracic surgery; he also introduced the very potent inhalational anaesthetic cyclopropane and the intravenous anaesthetic thiopental (Pentothal). Of even more importance, he set very high standards of clinical care and instituted regular meetings where all his staff reviewed the complications and deaths associated with anaesthesia. This degree of intellectual honesty was unusual at that time, for those in private practice could not afford to publicize the complications encountered in their practice. Waters later expanded his teaching and research programmes, which became internationally recognized and copied worldwide.[3,4]

Waters did not approve of nurse–anesthetists, though he did not actively oppose their employment as did McMechan. It is not surprising,

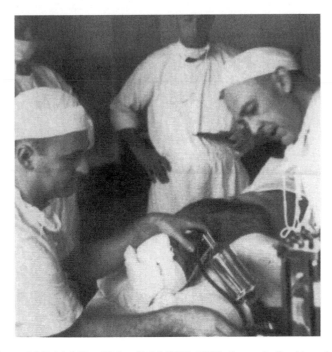

Figure 4.2 Ralph Milton Waters (right) (1883–1979), demonstrating his carbon dioxide absorption apparatus to a student when he visited John Lundy to learn regional anaesthesia in 1926. (Reproduced from Rehder K, Southorn P, Sessler A. *Art to Science, Department of Anesthesiology Mayo Clinic*. Rochester, MN: Mayo Clinic, 2000: 26. By permission of Mayo Foundation for Medical Education and Research. All rights reserved.)

therefore, that one of Waters's first trainees, Emery A Rovenstine, gradually weaned the surgeons from nurse to physician anaesthesia when he moved to the Bellevue Hospital in New York in 1935.[5] Rovenstine was also an inspired teacher, and was a great proponent of the use of local anaesthetic nerve blocks for the treatment of chronic pain. He became the second American professor of anesthesiology in 1937, had a major influence on the development of anaesthesia in the USA, and trained many anaesthetists from the USA and elsewhere (Figure 4.3). Many of Waters's other trainees subsequently became heads of departments throughout the USA, and they in turn promulgated Waters's ideas. Waters's trainees call themselves the 'aqualumni' and still meet regularly in Madison to refresh their 'family' ties.

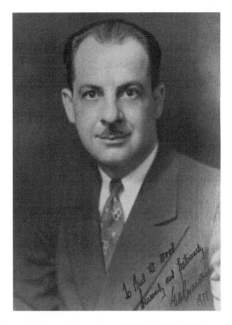

Figure 4.3 Emery Andrew Rovenstine (1895–1960), Bellevue Hospital, New York, the second professor of anaesthesia in the USA. (Reproduced with kind permission from Wood Library–Museum of Anesthesiology, Park Ridge, Illinois.)

Henry Knowles Beecher

In Boston, as always, things were done differently – in 1936, they appointed a surgeon to the post of Anesthetist-in-Chief in the Division of Surgery and Instructor of Anesthesia at Harvard. True, the man they appointed, Henry Knowles Beecher, had graduated *cum laude* in 1932, had trained for two years as a surgeon in Edward Churchill's department at the Massachusetts General Hospital, and had then worked in Nobel Laureate August Krogh's physiology laboratory in Copenhagen. But – and it was very big 'but' – he had not received any formal training in anaesthesia. Beecher responded to the challenge by teaching himself how to give anaesthetics, by writing a textbook on *The Physiology of Anaesthesia*, and by introducing the basic principles of laboratory research to the clinical practice of anaesthesia. His efforts were rewarded when he was appointed Henry Isaiah Dorr Professor of Research and

Teaching in Anaesthetics and Anaesthesia, a Chair that had been funded originally in 1917. In 1941, he thus became the first incumbent of the first Chair to be endowed in anaesthesia (Figure 4.4).

Beecher had a distinguished wartime career studying pain and shock in wounded men, as recounted in Chapter 7. In his academic career following the war, he is perhaps best known among anaesthetists and surgeons for his attempts to quantify pain and the action of analgesic drugs, for the study of the role of anaesthetic drugs in surgical mortality (the 'Beecher and Todd study' discussed in Chapter 10), and for his seminal studies of acid–base balance and respiratory acidosis during anaesthesia for thoracic surgery. He is remembered today worldwide for his tireless crusade to introduce ethical principles into clinical research and for his leadership in establishing the criteria for the diagnosis of brain death as the basis for the transplantation of human organs.[6]

Other contributors to the academic development of anaesthesia in the USA

There were a number of other anaesthetists who were not university professors but who nevertheless made major contributions to the

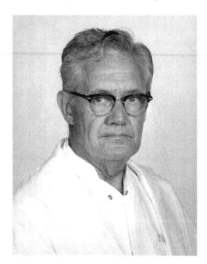

Figure 4.4 Henry Knowles Beecher (1904–76), Henry Isaiah Dorr Professor of Anaesthesia, Harvard Medical School, Boston. (Reproduced with the permission of the Department of Anesthesia, Massachusetts General Hospital.)

development of academic anaesthesia. One such was John Silas Lundy, Head of Anaesthesia at the Mayo Clinic in Rochester from 1924 until he was mysteriously ousted in 1952.[1,2] Lundy was born in 1894 in the Dakota Territories, and qualified as a physician in 1920. After an internship in Detroit, he moved to Seattle and started to practise anaesthesia. Although he had no formal training, he soon built up a lucrative practice and was elected Secretary of the King County Medical Society in 1924. In that year, Will Mayo, one of the two brothers who had founded the Mayo Clinic, lectured to the Society, and Lundy arranged to sit opposite him at the annual dinner. Lundy's enthusiasm for the recently introduced inhalation anaesthetic ethylene so impressed Mayo that he offered him a post in Rochester. Within a few weeks, Lundy had moved to the Mayo Clinic, where he found that he was designated head of the section on regional anaesthesia (Figure 4.5). He found that he was the only doctor interested in anaesthesia, and that most of the anaesthetics (mostly open-drop ether), were being given by 18 nurse–anesthetists.

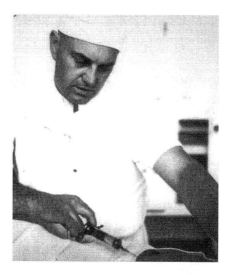

Figure 4.5 John Silas Lundy (1893–1973), Head of Department of Anesthesiology, Mayo Clinic, Rochester, Minnesota administering intravenous anaesthesia. (Reproduced from Rehder K, Southorn P, Sessler A. *Art to Science, Department of Anesthesiology Mayo Clinic*. Rochester, MN: Mayo Clinic, 2000: 23. By permission of Mayo Foundation for Medical Education and Research. All rights reserved).

Gaston Labat, a surgeon from Paris, had spent a year furthering an interest in local anaesthesia at the Mayo Clinic, so Lundy initially concentrated on the use of local anaesthetic agents and soon became very skilled in their use. As mentioned above, in 1926, Ralph Waters spent three months with him learning these techniques. Over the ensuing 25 years, Lundy developed a department with an international reputation, and many of his trainees became heads of departments elsewhere. Lundy spearheaded a number of advances. In 1926, he put forward the idea of using 'balanced anaesthesia' – the combined use of a number of different agents such as premedication, regional anaesthesia and light general anaesthesia to reduce the complications associated with deep general anaesthesia.[7] He was one of the first anaesthetists to investigate the use of the barbiturate drugs in anaesthesia. He tried sodium amytal in 1929 and sodium pentobarbital (Nembutal) in 1930, but both these agents had prolonged recovery times. He used hexobarbital (Evipan) in 1932, and started to investigate the use of thiopental in 1934, but was pre-empted by Ralph Waters, who published his early experiences with the drug in that year.

In 1933, the anaesthetists at St Mary's Hospital in Rochester applied their expertise in venepuncture to provide blood transfusions in children, and in the following year they assumed this responsibility in adults. At that time, the donor had to be present at the time of transfusion, but by the following year, Lundy reported that they had frequently kept citrated blood for up to 14 days in the ice-box at the Mayo Clinic. This was a revolutionary development that transformed blood transfusion therapy. In 1942, Lundy described how they had developed a post-anaesthesia recovery room at St Mary's Hospital. This ensured that the unconscious patient could be carefully supervised by properly trained staff and was not subjected to the variable standard of care on the general wards. Although the benefits were obvious, most general hospitals did not start to develop similar wards until the 1950s or later. Finally, we should record that Dr Lundy played a prominent role in establishing various national organizations. The first of these was the Anesthetist's Travel Club, a small group of leading anaesthetists from the USA and Canada that first met in Rochester in 1929. In 1952, it became the Academy of Anesthesiology, an institution that has done much to advance the cause of academic anaesthesia. The second was the American Board of Anesthesiology, the organization responsible for developing and maintaining the standards of anaesthesia, and the third was the founding of the journal *Anesthesiology*, now the premier American anaesthetic journal. So, although Lundy never held the title of professor, he contributed enormously to the academic advancement of anaesthesia.

As we shall see in the next chapter, the University of Oxford displayed its own characteristic opposition to change.

References

1. Volpitto PP, Vandam LD, eds. The genesis of contemporary American anesthesiology, Springfield, IL: Charles C Thomas, 1982.
2. Rehder K, Southorn P, Sessler A. *Art to Science. Department of Anesthesiology, Mayo Clinic.* Rochester MN: Mayo Clinic, 2000.
3. Waters RM. The development of anesthesiology in the United States. *Journal of History of Medicine and Allied Sciences* 1946;**1**:595–606.
4. Morris LE, Schroeder ME, Warner ME, eds. *Ralph Milton Waters, MD: Mentor to a Profession.* Chicago: Wood Library–Museum of Anesthesiology, 2004.
5. Maltby JR. *Notable Names in Anaesthesia.* London: Royal Society of Medicine Press, 2002: 180.
6. A definition of irreversible coma. Report of the Ad Hoc Committee of the Harvard Medical School to examine the definition of brain death. *Journal of the American Medical Association* 1968;**205**:37–40.
7. Lundy JS. Balanced anesthesia. *Minnesota Medicine* 1926;**9**:399–404.

5 The Morris Motor Company and the origins of academic anaesthesia in the UK

In the UK, new developments often originate in a golf club, and the idea of creating an academic department of anaesthesia was no exception. In this case, the principal players were the car manufacturer William Morris, later Lord Nuffield, and a young New Zealand anaesthetist, Robert Reynolds Macintosh. When Nuffield offered to provide money for the creation of a Postgraduate Medical School at Oxford in 1936, the University initially refused to create a Chair in Anaesthetics because it did not consider that anaesthesia was an academic subject. The University officials eventually relented, and Robert Reynolds Macintosh became the first Nuffield Professor of Anaesthetics. This appointment was to have a major impact on the development of anaesthesia throughout the world.

William Morris and the Oxford Chair

William Morris came from humble stock. He was born in Worcestershire in 1877, the son of a farm labourer. The family moved to Oxford, but his father became ill, so, at the age of 15, William started to repair bicycles to augment the family income. He then built a cycle for a rather large local vicar, who used it to make a daily progress around his parish. The strength of the 27-inch frame obviously impressed potential customers, and he soon had a full order book. He gained additional publicity by competing in local cycle races, and by 1901 he was the cycling champion of Oxfordshire, Berkshire and Buckinghamshire. The cycle business expanded rapidly, and, in 1901, he obtained a contract to repair all the bicycles used by the Oxford Post Office telegraph boys, and moved into premises in the High Street. His mechanical expertise was much in demand when the first motorcycles and cars appeared in Oxford, and he soon created a thriving car sales and repair business.[1]

Within a short time, Morris had switched to the assembly of cars from bought-in parts, the first two-seater 'Bullnose' Morris car being advertised at the 1912 motor show, although the first model was not actually produced until 1913 (Figure 5.1). In 1913, he sold 393 Morris Oxford cars at a price of £175 each, and in the next year 909 cars were sold. The factory at Cowley (near Oxford) was then switched to the manufacture of shell cases and mine sinkers for the duration of the war. After the war, there was a huge

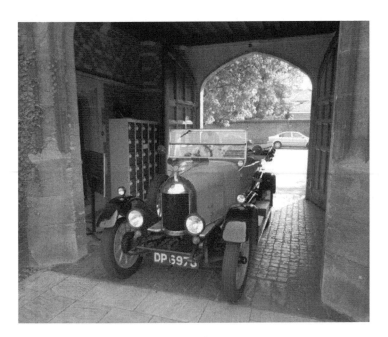

Figure 5.1 A 1925 Four-Seater Morris Cowley Tourer, owned by Chris Lovelock of The Bullnose Morris Club, entering the archway into Wantage Hall, University of Reading, on the Club's 2005 Autumn Rally. At the 1912 motor show, Morris advertised the Bullnose as 'the car that does 50 miles an hour and 50 miles to the gallon. Price £175'. By 1925, Morris was making 52 000 cars a year, commanding over 40% of the British market. (Reproduced by kind permission of Dr Peter McWilliam, Editor of the *Bullnose Morris Club Magazine* and Mr Chris Lovelock.)

expansion of the manufacturing facilities at Cowley, and by 1925 Morris had broken the monopoly of the Model T Ford and was selling over 50 000 cars a year. In 1927, Morris turned down an offer of 11 million pounds from General Motors when they tried to purchase the business.

Morris was very much a loner and, while loyal to his workforce, often bore a grudge against certain people and institutions. At the beginning of the century, he had a brief but disastrous commercial partnership with a rich undergraduate that set him against the University, and for many years he would not employ graduates in his organization. He also had many battles with the City Council over their refusal to update the old horsedrawn bus service. Eventually, he started a rival motorbus service, which he then sold to the Council. He twice refused the Freedom of the City, and only accepted it when the original members who opposed him over the bus issue had retired.

Morris was always interested in social problems and in medicine, and in 1926 he gave £10 000 to enable parents to visit their children in Borstal (corrective) institutions.[2] He recognized that British exports to Spain and South America were being hindered by a lack of knowledge of the language, and gave a similar sum to the University of Oxford to found the King Alphonso XIII Chair of Spanish Studies. These benefactions were soon followed by donations to hospitals in Birmingham and Coventry (where he had factories) and to St Thomas's Hospital in London. In the 1930s, he made donations for the rebuilding of the Radcliffe Infirmary and the Oxford Orthopaedic Hospital (which became the Wingfield–Morris Orthopaedic Hospital). He also provided funds for the purchase of the old University Observatory site, part of which was later used for the expansion of the Radcliffe Infirmary. The Observatory itself was used to house the Nuffield Institute of Medical Research, where Geoffrey Dawes later unravelled the changes in the fetal circulation at birth. The Observatory has now become part of Green College. Morris was knighted in 1929 and raised to the peerage in 1934. He chose the name of the village in which he lived for his title, and thus became Lord Nuffield (Figure 5.2).

Huntercombe Golf Club and the Nuffield Benefaction

Morris's main recreation was golf, and in 1927 he purchased Huntercombe Golf Club, a rather exclusive club near Henley, which was having financial difficulties. A number of doctors from Guy's Hospital and their wives frequented this club, and the New Zealand anaesthetist Robert Reynolds Macintosh and his wife Marjorie were amongst them. Morris often used to dine at the common table at the golf club, and discussed possible medical benefactions with the Guy's consultants.[3]

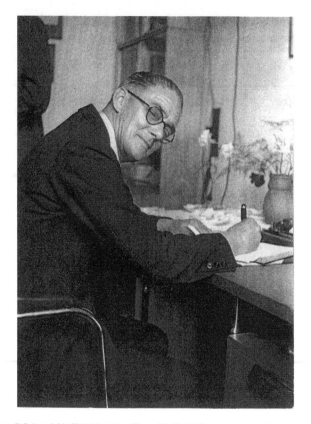

Figure 5.2 Lord Nuffield in his office. (Nuffield Department of Anaesthetics, Oxford.)

In 1936, Nuffield listened to a speech by Sir Farquhar Buzzard, Regius Professor of Medicine, at the British Medical Association Annual Meeting in Oxford. Buzzard had put forward the idea of a postgraduate medical school in Oxford, a concept that mirrored Nuffield's own ideas. (The Postgraduate Medical School at Hammersmith Hospital in London had been founded the previous year, but at that time there was some doubt about its potential.) Shortly after this meeting, Nuffield told his medical friends that he proposed to donate money to the University of Oxford to establish chairs of medicine, surgery, and obstetrics and gynaecology (the usual triumvirate that held a dominant position in most medical schools). To break the silence after this stunning announcement, Macintosh casually joked that anaesthetics had been left out again. Little further was said at the time, but doubtless Nuffield would have recalled the difference between his own early experiences of the crude nitrous oxide anaesthetics given by his dentist and the much more pleasant experience of an intravenous anaesthetic given by Macintosh. Whatever the stimulus, Nuffield decided to add a chair of anaesthetics to his proposal.

Given the state of anaesthesia at the time, it is not surprising that the University opposed the idea of a chair and suggested that the post should be downgraded to a Readership (Associate Professorship). Nuffield is quoted as saying that he was aware of the problem and recognized that it would take three generations before the subject could attain scientific credibility, but it was a chair or nothing. Finally, the University relented, and not only created the chair, but also appointed Macintosh to it. Subsequently, Nuffield increased his benefaction from 1.25 to 2 million pounds. The postgraduate medical school was founded, but was almost immediately overtaken by the exigencies of war, which resulted in many medical students being evacuated to Oxford for clinical training. This ultimately led to the development of the large clinical school that exists today. However, Macintosh believed that this development was contrary to Nuffield's intention to create a postgraduate institution, and, as a mark of protest, he never wore a gown on University occasions. Such was his loyalty to Nuffield.

Robert Reynolds Macintosh

So who was Macintosh? He was born at Timaru, a small town situated between Christchurch and Dunedin in the South Island of New Zealand, on 17 October 1897.[4,5] He was thus 10 years younger than Nuffield. His father was Charles Nicholson Macintosh, who played in the first New Zealand rugby team to tour Australia in 1893, and who was Mayor of Timaru in 1901 and 1902. Shortly afterwards, the family migrated to South America, where Macintosh senior edited a newspaper and speculated in land. Macintosh's father, brother and sister remained in South America, but he returned to New Zealand with his mother when he was 13 years old. His mother died shortly after their return, and he was sent to Waitaki Boys' High School, where he shone academically and athletically and was Head of School. In December 1915, he sailed to England and was commissioned in the Royal Scots Fusiliers. After a short period in France, he was transferred to the Royal Flying Corps, for which he had originally volunteered. He was mentioned in dispatches, but was shot down by the German ace Paul Strähle on 22 May 1917. He was not injured and managed to blow up his plane before being taken prisoner. There followed a remarkable series of escapes from various prisoner-of-war camps, but he never managed to cross the German border.[6]

After the war, Macintosh entered Guy's Hospital Medical School, qualifying MRCS, LRCP in 1924. He started to train as a surgeon and financed his studies by undertaking dental anaesthesia sessions in the Guy's Dental School, and although he obtained the Edinburgh FRCS in 1927, he found that the dental surgeons were increasingly employing him in their private practice. He soon built up a lucrative Harley Street practice with WS O'Connell, later Senior Anaesthetist at Guy's Hospital, and Bernard Johnson, later Senior Anaesthetist at the Middlesex Hospital. The group was highly organized, each doctor being assisted by a technician who drove the car, set up the apparatus, and then assisted the anaesthetist in the dental surgery or nursing home. One of these men was Richard Salt, who became the Chief Workshop Technician at Oxford, and subsequently played a major role in the development of the curved blade of the Macintosh laryngoscope, the various Oxford vaporizers, single- and double-lumen tracheal tubes, and countless other devices. The anaesthetists who were in competition with this practice, and whose rooms were heated by fuel supplied by the lorries of The Mayfair Gas, Light and Coke Company, rechristened the practice 'The Mayfair Gas, Fight and Choke Company' – or Mayfair Gas Company for short – a telling reference to the difficulties of inducing and maintaining a suitable level of anaesthesia with nitrous oxide.

Macintosh had visited Ralph Waters at the University of Wisconsin in the early 1930s and greatly admired his methods. Waters had three priorities: a high standard of clinical care, the teaching of medical students and trainees, and the prosecution of research. When Macintosh took up his post in 1937, he attempted to follow these precepts but found that the basic scientists were not prepared to cooperate in research. The reason was that many of the basic science departments feared that the new medical school would be a drain on scarce University funds.[7]

Wartime research

Macintosh soon made an impact, however. He discovered that in England there were only seven iron lung ventilators for treating poliomyelitis, and persuaded Lord Nuffield to manufacture 800 more, using a simplified design originated by Ted Both, an Australian engineer who was visiting Britain at the time of the 1937 polio epidemic (Figure 5.3). In 1938,

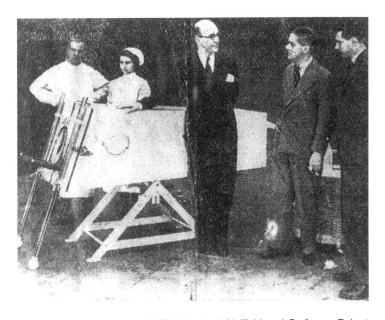

Figure 5.3 *(Right to left)* Mr ET Both, Lord Nuffield and Professor Robert Macintosh standing by one of the Both ventilators made in the Morris works at Cowley, Oxford. (Nuffield Department of Anaesthetics, Oxford.)

Macintosh spent six weeks in Spain anaesthetizing for an American plastic surgeon, Eastman Sheehan, who was operating on casualties from the Civil War. The only anaesthetic apparatus in the hospital was an outdated French vaporizer, so Macintosh improvised his own 'Flagg can' (Figure 5.4). This experience made him realize that there was great need for a simple vaporizer that could deliver known concentrations of ether in air under field conditions. With the cooperation of physicists from the Clarendon Laboratory, the Oxford Vaporizer No.1 was produced in 1941 (Figure 5.5). Some 2700 of these vaporizers were manufactured in the Morris works in Cowley, near Oxford, and used throughout the war and the postwar period (Figure 5.6). Another invention was the curved blade of the Macintosh laryngoscope that greatly facilitated visualization of the larynx (see Figure 3.8(b) in Chapter 3). Because the blade lifted the base of the tongue rather than the epiglottis itself, it was less likely to produce reflex closure of the vocal cords, and so could be used under lighter levels of anaesthesia.[8]

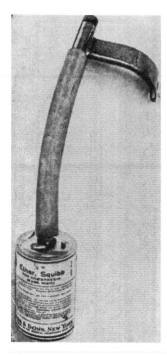

Figure 5.4 Flagg can. The patient breathed in and out over the ether in the can. The concentration of vapour was increased by swirling the ether around and warming the can with the hand. (Reproduced with kind permission from the Association of Anaesthetists of Great Britain and Ireland from Thomas KB. *The Development of Anaesthetic Apparatus*. Oxford: Blackwell Scientific, 1975.)

At the beginning of the Second World War Macintosh joined the RAF (Figure 5.7), but retained his connections with the Oxford department. He gathered together a team of doctors who were based in the department and who made a series of investigations that were of direct relevance to the war effort. One group investigated the physiological problems involved in escape from submarines (a problem posed by the recent *Thetis* disaster). Another group performed a series of hazardous experiments that involved the breathing of very low oxygen concentrations to simulate the descent of an airman from high altitude. These showed that survival was unlikely if the airman baled out above 35 000 feet without oxygen. One of those who participated in these

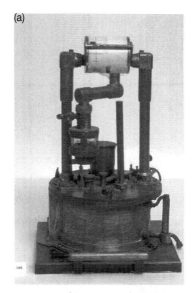

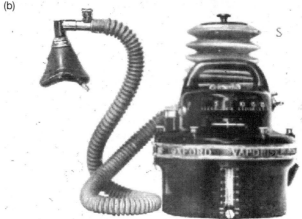

Figure 5.5 Oxford Vaporizer No 1: (a) prototype, 1940; (b) production model, 1941. Hot water was poured into the outer chamber. This melted the calcium chloride in the middle chamber. The melted calcium chloride provided heat to the inner ether chamber and maintained a constant temperature while changing back to the solid state. This enabled a constant concentration of ether to be maintained in the vaporizing chamber. The delivered concentration was controlled by varying the proportion of air that bypassed this chamber. (Nuffield Department of Anaesthetics, Oxford.)

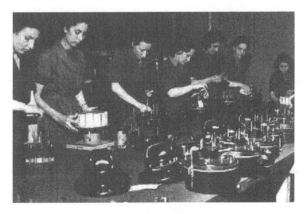

Figure 5.6 Wartime production line of Oxford vaporizers at the Morris Motor Works at Cowley, Oxford. (Nuffield Department of Anaesthetics, Oxford.)

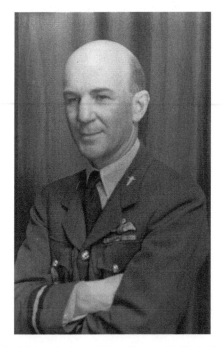

Figure 5.7 Robert Macintosh in RAF uniform with First World War wings (1943). (Reproduced by the kind permission of Mr Guy Francis, Oxford.)

experiments, the young anaesthetist Edgar A Pask (Figure 5.8), went on to perform even more remarkable studies. He had joined the Royal Air Force Aviation Institute in Farnborough and had found that airmen who had baled out over the North Sea were dying because their life-jackets turned them face down. Since there were no anthropomorphic models at that time, he decided that the only way to test new designs was to have Macintosh anaesthetize him deeply with ether and then to be thrown into a swimming pool wearing the jacket under test (Figure 5.9). During the course of these experiments, 17 life-jackets were tested, the final tests being performed in a pool at Ealing studios where there was a wave-making machine. As Macintosh later said '*Pask must be the only person to have gathered material for his MD thesis while deeply anaesthetised with ether*'.[9]

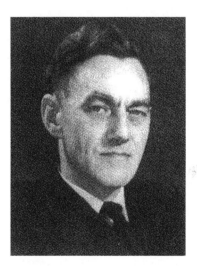

Figure 5.8 Professor Edgar Alan Pask OBE (1912–66). In 1941, he joined the Royal Air Force and conducted research into escape from aircraft at high altitudes, methods of artificial respiration, and development of survival suits and life-jackets, all at great personal risk to himself. He also designed an oxygen mask that allowed Churchill to smoke his cigar while flying to Moscow, but Churchill was not pleased, because his cigar burnt fiercely in the oxygen-enriched atmosphere. After the war, Pask spent some time in Ralph Waters's department in Madison, and became Reader in Anaesthetics at the University of Newcastle in 1947 and Professor in 1948. He was an innovative scientist, who maintained the highest standards and was greatly respected by all who knew him. (Nuffield Department of Anaesthetics, Oxford.)

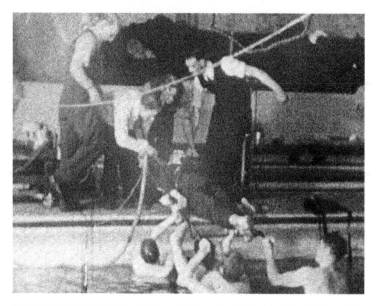

Figure 5.9 The anaesthetized Squadron Leader EA Pask testing life-jackets in a swimming pool. Professor Macintosh is standing on the left and the Chief Technician, Richard Salt, is next to him. (Still from the film recording the event, Nuffield Department of Anaesthetics, Oxford.)

But perhaps the most important contribution that the department made throughout the war was to run two-week courses on anaesthesia for doctors from the UK and overseas. Members of the department taught simple, safe techniques of anaesthesia that were applicable in any situation: they thus helped to remedy the severe shortage of anaesthetists during the war.

Postwar travels

After the war, Macintosh found that the promised accommodation for the Nuffield department had still not materialized, so he began to accept invitations to lecture and demonstrate anaesthesia in other parts of the world. He took with him an EMO (Epstein*–Macintosh–Oxford)

* RM Epstein was a physicist who had left Germany before the war. He was responsible for much of the design and testing of a series of Oxford vaporizers. He was also a coauthor with Macintosh and Mushin of the second edition of the book *Physics for the Anaesthetist*, first published in 1946. This book showed that a knowledge of physics was essential for the anaesthetist.

vaporizer (a later version of the Oxford ether vaporizer), an Oxford inflating bellows, some tracheal tubes, a Macintosh laryngoscope and some intravenous drugs such as thiopental and curare, and with these simple tools he coped with a wide range of operations (Figure 5.10). In most of the countries that he visited, anaesthesia was in a primitive state and limited to open-drop ether or spinal anaesthesia, so his demonstrations of the benefits of light ether anaesthesia combined with muscle relaxants were a revelation to many surgeons and potential anaesthetists (Figure 5.11). Macintosh's visits stimulated many anaesthetists to gain further experience abroad, and in the two decades after the war a large number of these anaesthetists either attended the British Council-funded courses on anaesthesia in Britain or gained experience in British anaesthetic departments.[10] Macintosh was knighted in 1955, retired in 1965 and died in 1989.

A personal note (Keith Sykes)

Robert Macintosh was the first Nuffield Professor of Anaesthetics, and was succeeded in 1965 by Alex Crampton Smith, who had been a Consultant in the department (Figure 5.12). When I was invited to become the third occupant of the chair in 1980, I recalled that, in 1936,

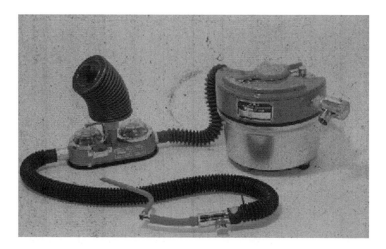

Figure 5.10 EMO (Epstein–Macintosh–Oxford) vaporizer with an Oxford inflating bellows connected to a tracheal tube. Macintosh travelled the world demonstrating that safe and effective anaesthesia could be produced with this simple apparatus. (Nuffield Department of Anaesthetics, Oxford.)

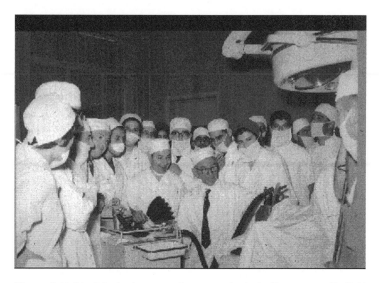

Figure 5.11 Macintosh demonstrating anaesthesia in Damascus. (Nuffield Department of Anaesthetics, Oxford.)

Nuffield had said that there would have to be three generations of professors before anaesthesia could attain academic credibility. Since I had only achieved a third-class BA degree at Cambridge, had no higher degree, had never had any training in basic research and had only a modicum of training in clinical research, I was naturally apprehensive. Fortunately, my predecessor, Alex Crampton Smith, who had pioneered many of the early developments in the use of mechanical ventilation in the Oxford respiratory unit in the 1950s, had laid the foundations for future progress. There were well-equipped laboratories, two physicists, an electronics engineer, 25 University/NHS technicians, and ongoing research projects in lung and heart function. But the department had been without a professor for a year and had been split between the cosy confines of the old Radcliffe Infirmary and the new, but incomplete, John Radcliffe Hospital, and morale was low.

There followed a number of years of intense activity. Major financial support was obtained from the Medical Research Council, the Wellcome Trust, the British Heart Foundation, the Association of Anaesthetists, the *British Journal of Anaesthesia* and other charitable foundations, and within a few years we had some 20 full-time research fellows studying for higher degrees. Approximately half of these were anaesthetists,

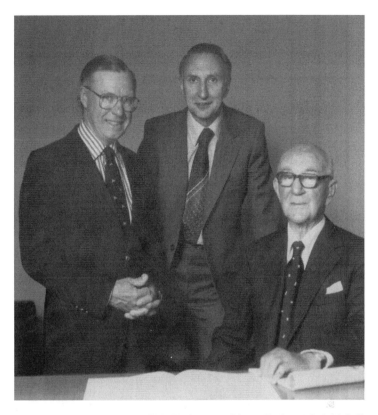

Figure 5.12 The first three Nuffield Professors of Anaesthetics at Oxford: *(left)* Alexander Crampton Smith (1965–89); *(centre)* Sir Keith Sykes (1989–91); *(right)* Sir Robert Macintosh (1937–65). (Nuffield Department of Anaesthetics, Oxford.)

cardiologists or doctors working in intensive care units, and the other half physiologists, pharmacologists, mathematicians, physicists or engineers. The latter group spent a third or more of their three-year period in research working in our laboratories on the applications of their science to anaesthesia, intensive care or pain relief. Whereas Macintosh had received a cool reception from the basic science departments, our proposals for cooperative research projects were welcomed; this enabled us to utilize the resources of a prestigious university. In return, we were able to contribute by lecturing to undergraduates in the basic science departments. But my transition from a clinical anaesthetist to a university professor was just one example of the way in which academic anaesthesia developed worldwide during the postwar period.

Academic anaesthesia in the postwar period

After the war, there was a major expansion of academic anaesthesia in the USA, the UK and many other countries in the world. In the USA, major departments were developed by Robert Dripps in Philadelphia and by Emmanuel Papper in New York to compliment the Madison and Boston departments, and these were followed by the creation of a number of other departments in other cities. In the UK, seven new departments of anaesthesia were created in 1947–48, and by 1968 there were 20 academic departments of anaesthesia, though not all were headed by a Professor.[11] Furthermore, a number of these departments were partially funded by the NHS because it was recognized that the presence of an academic department would stimulate trainees to enter the region, and so help to alleviate staffing shortages. Many of these departments developed significant research programmes, and thus contributed to the increased knowledge of the scientific basis of anaesthesia, intensive care and pain relief. It was the anaesthetists' knowledge of heart and lung function that established them as lead clinicians in intensive care.

But while the university departments were important, there were two other institutions that had a major impact on standards of practice.

The Faculty of Anaesthetists and the foundation of a Royal College

In 1932, a group of anaesthetists who were concerned with the poor standards of practice and the lowly status of the anaesthetist formed the Association of Anaesthetists of Great Britain and Ireland. The three main aims were to promote the development of anaesthesia; to represent anaesthetists and to promote their interests; and to favour the establishment of a Diploma in Anaesthetics.[12] The Diploma was strongly supported by Ivan Magill, of tracheal intubation and thoracic anaesthesia fame, and was initiated in 1935, but since the Association was not an examining body, the examination was run by the Conjoint Board of the Royal Colleges of Physicians and Surgeons.

The formation of the National Health Service (NHS) in 1948 provided a further stimulus to the academic development of anaesthesia. A number of leading anaesthetists (most of whom were actively involved with the Association) realized that the Diploma was no longer an adequate examination. If anaesthetists were to achieve and hold Consultant status in the NHS, it would be necessary to create a body similar to the Royal College of Surgeons that would be concerned primarily with academic standards in anaesthesia. The Council of the Association of Anaesthetists and the President of the Royal College of Surgeons actively supported this concept, and in 1948 a Faculty of Anaesthetists was created in the Royal College of Surgeons. The Faculty subsequently metamorphosed into an independent College of Anaesthetists, and the College was given Royal status in 1992. Shortly after its foundation, the Faculty took over the responsibility for the Diploma in Anaesthetics that had been initiated in 1935, and created a two-part examination with a standard equivalent to the Fellowship examinations of the other major Royal Colleges. The first part was initially modelled closely upon the Primary examination of the Royal College of Surgeons, with papers and *viva voce* examinations in the basic sciences of anatomy, physiology, pathology and pharmacology, while the second part covered clinical medicine and surgery and all the clinical aspects of anaesthesia.

In 1953, the examination was renamed the Fellowship of the Faculty of Anaesthetists of the Royal College of Surgeons (FFARCS) and the opportunity was taken to change the basic sciences examined in the first part to those more appropriate to anaesthesia (physiology, pharmacology, physics and clinical measurement). However, the standard has always been strictly comparable to that of the Fellowship examinations of the other Royal Colleges. Candidates for the Fellowship examinations of the Royal College of Anaesthetists (FRCA) know that they will be expected to have a detailed knowledge of the basic sciences related to anaesthesia as well as a broad knowledge of all aspects of internal medicine, anaesthesia, resuscitation, intensive care, and methods of relieving acute and chronic pain.

All British trainees now have to enrol in a carefully supervised seven-year training programme in one of the regional Schools of Anaesthesia associated with the university academic departments, and have to pass the FRCA examination before they are eligible to apply for a Consultant appointment in an NHS hospital. Nuffield would have been surprised and gratified had he seen the results of his two million pound donation to the reluctant University of Oxford.

References

1. Hull P. *Lord Nuffield 1877–1963. An Illustrated Life of William Richard Morris, Viscount Nuffield*, 2nd edn. Princes Risborough: Shire Publications, 1993.
2. Minns FJ, ed. *Wealth Well-Given: The Enterprise and Benevolence of Lord Nuffield*. Stroud, UK: Alan Sutton, 1994.

3. Beinart J. *A History of the Nuffield Department of Anaesthetics, Oxford 1937–87*. Oxford: Oxford University Press, 1987.

4. 'Macintosh RR'. In: Nicholls CS, ed. *The Dictionary of National Biography, 1986–1990*. Oxford: Oxford University Press, 1996.

5. Sykes M.K. Macintosh: from Timaru to Timbuktu. *Journal of the Scottish Society of Anaesthetists* 1995;**35**:9–14.

6. Hervey HE. *Cagebirds*. London: Penguin, 1940.

7. Sykes K. How Ralph Waters influenced the development of anaesthesia in the British Commonwealth and in Europe. In: Morris LE, Schroeder ME, Warner ME, eds. *Ralph Milton Waters, MD: Mentor to a Profession*. Park Ridge, IL: Wood Library–Museum of Anesthesiology, 2004: 192–204.

8. Bryce-Smith R. Mitchell JV, Parkhouse J, eds. *The Nuffield Department of Anaesthetics, Oxford 1937–62*. Oxford: Oxford University Press, 1963.

9. Obituary: Edgar Pask. *Lancet* 1966;**i**:1330–1.

10. Sykes K, Benad G. The influence of Sir Robert Reynolds Macintosh on the development of anaesthesia. *Anaesthesiologie und Reanimation* 2004;**29**:91–6.

11. Nunn J.F. Development of academic anaesthesia in the UK up to the end of 1998. *British Journal of Anaesthesia* 1999;**83**:916–32.

12. Boulton TB. *The Association of Anaesthetists of Great Britain and Ireland 1932–1992 and the Development of the Specialty of Anaesthesia*. London: Association of Anaesthetists of Great Britain and Ireland, 1999.

Further reading

Rushman GB, Davies NJH, Atkinson RS. *A Short History of Anaesthesia. The First 150 Years*. London: Butterworth–Heinemann, 1996:41–2.

Sykes K. Sir Robert Reynolds Macintosh. In: *Careers in Anaesthesiology*. Park Ridge, IL: Wood Library–Museum of Anesthesiology, 2005:35–65.

6 The impact of the Second World War

On 3 September 1939, as Hitler's tanks thundered into Poland, Britain declared war on Germany. On 7 December 1941, some 200 Japanese aircraft attacked the US Fleet anchored in Pearl Harbor, and the USA joined the Allied cause. In the ensuing conflict, there were many casualties among the civilian population and the Armed Forces, and anaesthetists often had to work under appalling conditions. However, the reorganization of medical services and the experience of anaesthetizing seriously ill casualties had a major beneficial impact on the future development of the specialty.

Anaesthesia for the armed services had received scant attention during the First World War. The few army doctors trained in anaesthesia were overwhelmed by the enormous number of casualties, and anaesthesia was provided by doctors when available, but more generally by medically unqualified personnel. We have already recounted in Chapter 3 how Arthur Guedel, one of the few trained anaesthetists among the American forces, drove by motorbike to guide and encourage the personnel working in the forward units, but he was unusual in having had extensive experience of anaesthesia.

In the period between the wars, a small but growing number of doctors started to practise anaesthesia full-time, but most of these worked in the teaching hospitals or in private practice.[1] In the UK, the majority of anaesthetics were given by general practitioners, house doctors, or even medical students or theatre porters, while in the USA, a large proportion of anaesthetics were given by nurse–anesthetists. The specialists in the USA initially called themselves 'physician–anesthetists', but, with the formation of professional societies and certification boards shortly before the USA entered the Second World War, they were renamed 'anesthesiologists', to distinguish them from nurse–anesthetists. The second American anesthetic journal, which was founded in 1940, was named *Anesthesiology*.[2]

In prewar Britain, an intravenous induction was usually only given by the specialist anaesthetist, and most patients were anaesthetized with ether or chloroform, often preceded by nitrous oxide or a rapidly acting volatile agent such as ethyl chloride or divinyl ether (Vinesthene). The latter agents were very potent and speeded up the induction, but were unpleasant to inhale and too volatile for prolonged use. In hospitals where there were no anaesthetists, the surgeon often gave a spinal anaesthetic or a regional nerve block, or infiltrated the tissues with local anaesthetic. Dental extractions were performed at great speed under a short nitrous oxide anaesthetic given by a dentist or general practitioner, with the patient strapped upright in a dental chair, and minor or emergency operations were often performed in the patient's home. It is not surprising that relatively few operations were performed, and that most of the operations outside the specialist hospitals were for common conditions such as hernia, tonsils and adenoids, or for emergency conditions such as bone fractures, appendicitis, perforated peptic ulcer and strangulated hernia.

But the war changed everything.

Emergency Medical Services

First, it changed the pattern of medical practice. While the general practitioners who were not called up for military service continued to practise from their surgeries, the civilian hospitals were reorganized on a regional basis to produce an Emergency Medical Service (EMS). This was designed to provide a large number of emergency beds for the immediate care of civilian air-raid casualties by removing routine and convalescent patients to more peripheral hospitals in safer areas (Figure 6.1). After the war, the EMS provided the basic hospital structure for the future National Health Service (NHS). The increase in trauma cases made it necessary to recruit salaried anaesthetists for the EMS hospitals, and many older general practitioner anaesthetists and others exempt from military service took up full-time anaesthetic posts in these hospitals. They often had to cope with an enormous load of surgical cases, and gained extensive experience of anaesthesia for many types of surgery that they would not have otherwise encountered. In Addenbrooke's Hospital in Cambridge, and in some other hospitals, nurses were employed to sustain the anaesthetic service, and during the blitz in Liverpool, a motor engineer, JH Blease, who had made some equipment for a local anaesthetist, helped his medical colleague in the operating

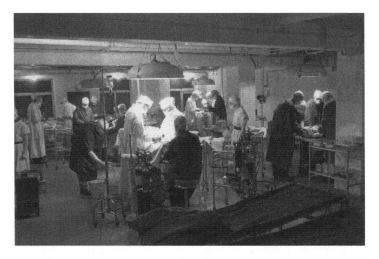

Figure 6.1 Operating theatre with four surgical teams working simultaneously at Guy's Hospital, London during the Second World War. (Photograph courtesy of the Imperial War Museum, London, Negative No. D2328.)

theatre. He decided that providing controlled ventilation by manual compression of a reservoir bag was rather boring and developed a mechanical bag-squeezer. This led him to set up in business as a manufacturer of mechanical ventilators and anaesthetic machines.

Another important development was that the Medical Research Council created three vital civilian organizations that persisted into the postwar period and became part of the new NHS. These were the Public Health Laboratory Service, the Hospital Laboratory Service and the Civilian Blood Transfusion Service. These played a vital role in medical care during and after the war.

The UK Armed Forces

A major reorganization also occurred in the UK Armed Forces. The Army, and to a lesser extent the other two Services, created a number of surgical teams with surgeons, anaesthetists, nursing and ancillary staff.[1] These teams worked together in forward positions and in base hospitals, and soon learnt how to resuscitate and sort casualties into priorities for surgery ('triage'). They learnt how to anaesthetize and operate on patients with severe wounds of the head, chest, abdomen or limbs, and thus performed the type of major surgical procedures that only the specialist would have attempted prewar. Blood banks were set up to provide blood and plasma for the recently introduced technique of blood transfusion, and doctors were trained to identify blood groups and to match the donor blood to that of the recipient. They also learnt how to treat shock by the transfusion of fluids, plasma and blood, and how to care for patients after operation. Such teamwork was almost unheard of in civilian practice at that time, and the experience gained was later to prove invaluable when these doctors, nurses and technicians returned to civilian life and became part of the NHS in 1948. It also created a team spirit that transformed relationships between the various specialities – a spirit that was later nurtured when these young specialists returned to work in NHS hospitals. This accounts for the fact that most British anaesthetists undertake regular clinical sessions with the same few surgeons with whom they develop a close rapport, whereas in most overseas departments, there is a more random allocation of anaesthetic staff to different surgical services.

The war also had a major impact on the development of anaesthesia in the USA, which entered the war after the disaster of Pearl Harbor.[2,3] On 7 December 1941, some 200 Japanese aircraft attacked the US Fleet anchored in Pearl Harbor. The USA suffered over 3400 casualties, 2300 of whom were killed (Figure 6.2). We have described in Chapter 3 how the medical staff, who had no experience of war and little knowledge of anaesthesia, used relatively large doses of thiopental as the sole anaesthetic agent for surgery, and how there were a number of deaths attributed to the anaesthetic.

In 1941, there were only a few departments in the USA offering training programmes for physicians, and there were no specialists in anaesthesia in the US Armed Forces. The immediate response was that a few departments, such as that at the Mayo Clinic, expanded their residency training programmes to generate more anaesthetists.[4] In addition, civilian doctors were rapidly inducted into the Army and Navy and enrolled in three-month training programmes, emerging as '90-day wonders'. Then, Ralph Tovell, who had created an active anaesthetic department at Hartford, Connecticut, was recruited into the US Army as a Lieutenant-Colonel to become Senior Consultant in Anesthesia.[5] There was no precedent for this appointment, but when Tovell was drafted to England, he met other anaesthetic consultants to the forces, such as Robert Macintosh (Royal Air Force), Ivan Magill (Royal Navy), Ashley Daley (British Army) and Beverly Leech (Canadian Army). Tovell set up special courses to train specialists for the armed services, and a significant number of anaesthetists from the USA and other allied countries attended short courses on anaesthesia at Oxford and other

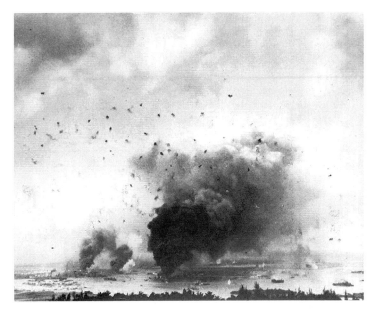

Figure 6.2 Japanese aerial photograph of Pearl Harbor under attack, 7 December 1941.

centres in the UK, or gained experience by being attached to British or American hospitals in the UK. Tovell also made a major contribution by harmonizing equipment standards so that British and American equipment could be used interchangeably. (At that time there were *five* different sizes of cone-and-socket joints used to connect the pipes to the various components in an anaesthetic breathing system – it is therefore not surprising that breathing circuits were sometimes wrongly assembled, often with disastrous results.)

Another American anaesthetist who distinguished himself during the war was Henry Beecher. He designed an anaesthetic machine that was used by the American forces, but, more importantly, he also carried out fundamental research on the problem of blood loss and surgical shock, and on the occurrence and relief of pain in wounded men.[6] The citation that accompanied the Award of the Legion of Merit summarized his accomplishments during this period:

> *'Colonel Beecher, by personally treating soldiers seriously*
> *wounded in combat, evolved principles and procedures of*

resuscitation and anesthesia that were accepted and put into practice in this and other theatres of war. First-hand experience gained during the cold winter months before Cassino and in the dugout, shock tents of the hospitals at Anzio was translated by him into basic concepts, to govern these phases of the management of the wounded soldier from the time the missile strikes until the damage it caused has been repaired. Original observations were made on the pain suffered by men wounded in battle that never had been recorded in the history of warfare, and combined with his observations on the hazards of the traditional use of morphine, those studies pointed the way toward the giving of this time honoured remedy on the battlefield in a way that was both safe and humane.'

We shall be discussing his work on pain in the next chapter.

The promise of peace

In the dark days of 1942, Sir William Beveridge published his report on 'Social Insurance and Allied Services' in which he outlined a blueprint for the future NHS in Britain. Beveridge stressed that his plan required '*a health service providing full preventative and curative treatment of every citizen without exception, and without an economic barrier at any point to delay recourse to it*'. Over the ensuing six years, the structure of the new NHS was fleshed out in innumerable meetings between the medical profession and government, but there was some doubt as to whether anaesthesia would be considered a speciality in its own right in the NHS. It was only after extensive discussions in 1947 that it was finally agreed that anaesthetists should be given speciality status comparable with the other branches of medicine in the NHS.[1] Now anaesthesia is one of the largest specialities in the NHS.

By the end of the war, medicine was a very different profession from that existing in the prewar period. There were a large number of relatively young but very experienced doctors who had learned how to work together under difficult circumstances and who were enthusiastic about a free health service. There were new treatments such as fluid and blood transfusion, and magical cures were being reported with the new wonder drug, penicillin.

Anaesthetists were now routinely inducing anaesthesia with thiopental, and curare was being used in a few leading centres, though it was being given in small doses so that some spontaneous respiration was preserved as a guide to dosage. At this time, anaesthetists usually *assisted* the patient's spontaneous breathing by compressing the reservoir bag in time with the patient's spontaneous breathing rhythm, but by the beginning of the 1950s, many anaesthetists were finding that they could provide superior operating conditions by employing larger doses of curare that completely paralysed the respiratory muscles. As a result, *controlled* ventilation became routine in major general surgery as well as in thoracic surgery. It was this type of ventilation that Bjørn Ibsen introduced when treating poliomyelitis in Copenhagen in 1952 (see Chapter 12).

Not surprisingly, a few of our more mechanically minded colleagues began to devise mechanical ventilators that could replace the anaesthetist's 'educated hand'. It was not until the late 1950s, however, that commercial versions of such machines began to appear in our operating theatres. Shortly afterwards, practical techniques for measuring the levels of oxygen and carbon dioxide in the blood were becoming available, so the anaesthetist could, at last, measure what was happening to the patient. It was the beginning of the scientific era of anaesthesia.

So, the Second World War, which left such devastation throughout many parts of the world, produced the conditions for the development of a new kind of medicine – one in which doctors began to apply science to their practice, and in which the advent of the antibiotics and other powerful drugs enabled doctors to cure diseases for the first time. Anaesthesia benefited more from the wartime experience than did most other branches of medicine, so anaesthetists were well placed to create a new pattern of anaesthetic practice that was firmly based on the emerging sciences of physiology, pharmacology, physics and clinical measurement. It was the foresight of those who reformed the academic curriculum in the postwar period that ultimately led the anaesthetist out of the operating room and into the sphere of acute medicine.

Before leaving our wartime story, we should examine one other field that benefited enormously from studies on the battlefield: the problem of pain and its treatment. This we do in the next chapter.

References

1. Boulton TB. *The Association of Anaesthetists of Great Britain and Ireland 1932–92 and the Development of the Speciality of Anaesthesia*. London: The Association of Anaesthetists of Great Britain and Ireland, 1999: 62–75.
2. Romanelli T, Bacon D. The origins of modern anesthesia throughout the American experience spanning the World Wars. *Bulletin of Anesthesia History* 1999;**17**:3–7.
3. Waisel DB. The role of World War II and the European Theater of Operations in the development of anesthesiology as a physician specialty in the USA. *Anesthesiology* 2001;**94**:907–14.

4. Lundy JS. Factors that influenced the development of anesthesiology. *Anesthesia and Analgesia* 1946;**25**:38–43.
5. Tovell RM. Problems of training in and practice of anesthesiology in the European Theater of Operations. *Anesthesiology* 1947;**8**:62–74.
6. Beecher HK. Anesthesia for men wounded in battle. *Annals of Surgery* 1945;**122**:807–19.

Further reading

Beecher HK. *Resuscitation and Anesthesia for Wounded Men. The Management of Traumatic Shock*. Springfield, IL: Charles C Thomas, 1949.

7 Henry Beecher, John Bonica and the treatment of pain

'We must all die, but that I can save him from days of torture, that is what I feel as my great and even new privilege. Pain is a more terrible lord of mankind than even death itself' (**Albert Schweitzer**)

The nature of pain

John Bonica, in his introduction to the groundbreaking textbook *The Management of Pain,*[1] wrote that *'The proper management of pain remains, after all, the most important obligation, the main objective, and the crowning achievement of* every *physician'*. While today this may be taken for granted, it was not always so. The benefits of the discovery of anaesthesia and the subsequent release from the agonies of surgically inflicted pain were by no means immediately recognized by the medical profession. There were not only justifiable initial concerns about the safety of anaesthetic agents, chloroform in particular, but valid medicolegal concerns as well:

> *'Nineteenth century American law offered few safeguards to medical researchers: physicians who did prescribe new drugs faced a real threat of prosecution. ... The Philadelphia* Medical Examiner *warned practitioners to consider "if fatal results should happen to one of their patients, what would be the effect upon their conscience, their reputation and business, and how the practice would be likely to be viewed by a Philadelphia court and jury" '.*[2]

In addition to such understandable concerns, it was also believed, apparently by many doctors, that pain was *'an essential part of the process of life, that the "annihilation of sensation itself impairs the health of the organs of the body", and "that anaesthesia, whatever its form, is an assault upon vital functions"'*.[2] Pain was equated not only with life in general, but was thought to be essential to the process of healing and the recovery from surgery. As noted in Chapters 20 and 21, the argument that pain is essential to the natural or normal progress of childbirth persists to this day.

Religious concerns also influenced the historical perceptions of the meaning of pain. A French historian explains that '*The* [Catholic] *Church has always had a dual system of explanation when it comes to physical pain: on the one hand, there has been the Augustian tradition which ... interprets pain as punishment for the wicked and a foretaste of the final retribution; and the other view which considers pain as a means of moral progression and salvation*'.[3] A century later, during what has been called a 'dolorist' trend between the two world wars, pain was considered '*a means of self-discovery ... [and] for a Christian could only be understood in terms of the final redemption and resurrection*'.[3]

Quite apart from any social or theological benefit attributed to pain, does it serve any biological purpose? Not much, argued the noted French surgeon Rene Leriche when confronted with the horror of pain during the First World War. Leriche wrote that pain '*reveals only a minute proportion of illnesses and often, when it is one of their accompaniments, it is misleading*'. But Leriche acknowledges that pain '*exists wherever there is life* [and that] *life cannot exist without it*'.[4] Pain does serve as an essential warning – to the doctor as well as to the patient. Just how important becomes dramatically apparent when one considers the medical catastrophes that may befall an individual in the absence of pain. The loss of fingers or toes, as frequently occurred in leprosy, was the direct result of the loss of sensation associated with the peripheral neuritis that occurs in that disease. With the affected person being unable to feel pain and to recognize injury or infection, the extremity may be so severely damaged or infected that it cannot be salvaged. The rare individual born without the ability to feel pain will sustain burns, bruises and lacerations. In the absence of pain, a ruptured appendix may not be recognized. Persons unable to feel pain die prematurely because of the effects of unrecognized trauma and subsequent infections.[5]

And finally, pain also serves an essential function during the recovery period from injury or infection, for it enforces rest in order to promote healing.

Pain in a time of war

Our understanding of the nature of pain owes much to observations of soldiers suffering wartime injuries. While the cause of acute pain suffered in battle seems obvious, the perception of that pain varies markedly from soldier to soldier. In his 1827 *Treatise on Gunshot Wounds*, GJ Guthrie, a British army surgeon, observed that '*in two persons suffering apparently from the same kind of injury, and with the same detriment, one will writhe with agony, whilst the other will smile with contempt*'.[6] The French surgeon Guillaume Dupuytren, known today primarily for having first described the contracture of the palm of the hand that bears his name, was quoted as saying '*What a difference there is in the morale of those we treat in civilian hospitals and those hit by murderous fire on the field of battle! He considers himself happy if he saves his life but loses an extremity* [and] *he faces with courage, even joy, the scalpel of the surgeon*'.[7]

During the Mexican/American War, which began in April 1846 (by coincidence the same year that surgical anaesthesia was introduced at the Massachusetts General Hospital), the Army surgeon John B Porter wrote that '*manly heroism, tempered in the fire of military life and honed by the excitement of battle, made soldiers insensitive to the pain of almost any operation*'.[8] A century later, in the Second World War, the absence of acute pain in wounded soldiers was confirmed by Henry Beecher (Figure 7.1). In the course of his duties as Consultant in Anesthesia and

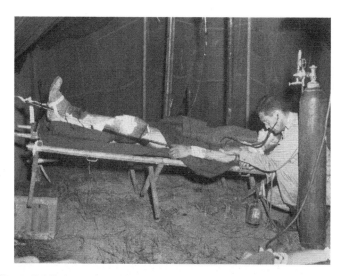

Figure 7.1 Dr Henry K Beecher in the shock tent at the Anzio beachhead. (Reproduced with permission from Beecher HK. *Resuscitation and Anaesthesia for Wounded Men*. Springfield, IL: Charles C Thomas, 1949.)

Resuscitation in the Mediterranean Theater of Operations, Beecher had the opportunity to make careful records of the extent of pain suffered by freshly wounded soldiers in the combat zone. He found that three-quarters of the badly wounded men rejected offers of pain medication. (This was despite the fact that none of them had received morphine for four hours, and many had received none at all, while none were in shock). He concluded that there was no dependable relation between the extent of a pathological wound and the pain experienced.[9]

Beecher observed that while many severely wounded soldiers, even though alert mentally and with normal blood pressure, do not complain of severe pain, most hospital patients following major surgery with wounds of equivalent severity complain bitterly of their wound pain. Beecher thought that their different responses were due to differences in the significance of pain to the soldier and to the civilian patient. He suggested that this represented a 'clinical' validation of the hypothesis, proposed more than a half century earlier by the philosopher and psychologist HR Marshall, that suffering consists of two principal factors: the initial sensation and the psychic reaction, or subjective response.[10]

The aftermath of battlefield injury and the treatment of chronic pain

The type and severity of injury also play a role in the incidence and severity of painful sequelae. Beecher made his observations on severely wounded soldiers at a forward hospital on the Anzio beachhead during the Second World War, and he would not have known the outcome of their injuries following evacuation. It can be assumed that some would not have survived their wounds, that some would have recovered quickly and without disability, but that some would have suffered prolonged or permanent injury. Some of the soldiers had lost an extremity, and some had suffered injuries to the head, to the spinal cord or to peripheral nerves.

The nature of many such injuries was described during the American Civil War by the army surgeon Silas Weir Mitchell, and his account remains a definitive classic today. In an 1867 monograph, *United States Sanitary Commission Memoirs*, Mitchell described an injury to a soldier *'who was shot in the left arm by a bullet that entered just above the elbow, penetrated without touching the artery, and emerged through the belly of the biceps'*. Mitchell wrote *'on the second day the pain began. It was burning and darting. Sensation was lost or lessened in the limb, and that paralysis of motion came on in the hand and forearm. The pain was so severe that a touch anywhere, or shaking the bed, or a heavy step, caused it to increase*'.[11] For this condition, resulting from injuries to nerves in the arm or leg, Mitchell coined the word 'causalgia', from the Greek *kauson*, heat or burning, and *algos*, pain. The pain of causalgia can usually be interrupted with local anaesthetic drugs injected into tissues surrounding the injured nerve, but the pain and hypersensitivity may return as the anaesthetic wears off, and may persist for months and years.

While Beecher was assigned to a forward hospital, another young army anaesthetist, John Bonica, was sent to Madigan Army Hospital in Fort Lewis, Washington (Figure 7.2). It had 7770 beds and was then described as the largest army hospital in the world. In addition to his assignment to provide anaesthesia for operative surgery, he was placed in charge of pain control.[12] 'Madigan received wounded men from all

(a)

(b)

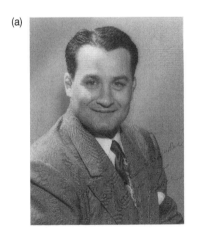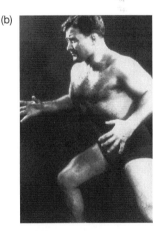

Figure 7.2 (a) John Joseph Bonica (1917–94), Professor and Chairman of the Anesthesiology Department at the University of Washington School of Medicine in Seattle, who originated the idea of multidisciplinary clinics for the treatment of chronic pain. (b) John Bonica was an Italian émigré who had to assume financial responsibility for his family when his father died in 1932. He took many different jobs to finance his studies, and paid his way through medical school by working as a professional wrestler during the vacations. He used names such as Johnny (Bull) Walker to avoid recognition by his medical colleagues, and was the light heavyweight champion of Canada in 1939 and World Champion in 1941. (Reproduced with kind permission from his daughter Angela Bonica DeSimone and the Wood Library–Museum of Anesthesiology, Park Ridge, Illinois.)

over the Pacific theater, many with puzzling intractable pain related to amputations or peripheral nerve injuries, a critical mass of unusual pain cases such as no civilian physician at that time would have been confronted.' Referring cases that he felt unable to manage to other specialists, Bonica found that they were equally at a loss. Although no one physician had the answer, he realized that each speciality brought a different and useful perspective to the diagnosis of intractable pain. Only by bringing together doctors from all of the relevant disciplines would it be possible to resolve many of the complex problems of chronic pain.

Bonica's new concept, the interdisciplinary approach to pain management, induced a fundamental shift in how we understand chronic pain today. From this beginning ultimately sprang the modern multidisciplinary pain clinic. Such clinics are now well established in North America and other English-speaking countries, and, to a lesser extent, in continental Europe. In Great Britain alone, the number of hospitals with a multidisciplinary pain clinic rose from fewer than 3% before 1990 to just under 50% in 1994, but there is still a wide variation in the geographical location of pain units and in the quality of care provided.

From clinical experience to a theory of pain

'Physical pain is not a simple affair of an impulse, travelling at a fixed rate along a nerve. It is the resultant of a compact between a stimulus and the whole individual.' (Rene Leriche)

Beecher's front-line observations in battle, and those of Guthrie and Porter in the previous century, focused on the relatively straightforward problem of acute pain. Bonica became responsible for the treatment of chronic pain that might be suffered for months and years in the aftermath. Their experiences stimulated laboratory studies that led to a gradual unravelling of the complex and multifaceted nature of pain. It became possible to construct a new theory to replace the earlier widely held assumption that there is a fixed, direct communication system from the skin to the brain, pain impulses being carried by nerve fibres in peripheral nerves and by specialized tracts in the spinal cord to a pain centre in the central nervous system.

The new theory, proposed in 1965 by the psychologist Ronald Melzack and the neurologist Patrick Wall, was called a 'physiological gate control system'.[13] It was suggested that the perception of pain reflects a balance between the sensory pain impulses arising from the periphery and centrally mediated inhibitory impulses. The theory emphasizes the importance of central mechanisms and portrays the brain as an active system that filters, selects and modulates neural inputs. It postulates that with persistent damage to peripheral nerves, notably in causalgia, phantom limb or peripheral neuralgia, the normal mechanisms that inhibit or modulate pain, that 'close the gate' to the perception of pain, become inoperative. That pain can exist in the brain or spinal cord independent of nervous input from the periphery is most dramatically evident following loss of an arm or leg. The missing extremity or 'phantom limb' may be perceived as still being present by the individual, and is frequently accompanied by severe and unremitting pain.

Beecher's observations of the lack of correlation between the physiological and psychological aspects of pain have been supported by other observations. For example, after lobotomy (the cutting of nervous tracts leading to the brain's frontal lobes, the site of emotional responses), patients report that they still have pain, but that it no longer bothers them. Patients in pain who receive morphine may state that they still feel pain but that their suffering has been relieved. And, finally, in Pavlov's famous studies of conditioned responses, dogs subjected to electric shocks, burns or cuts, and then presented with food, eventually responded to these stimuli as signals for food and failed to show 'even the tiniest and most subtle' signs of pain.

The publication of the gate control theory immediately provided a rationale for the multidisciplinary clinical approach advocated by Bonica. As Melzack commented, Bonica:

'had been trying valiantly to convince his medical colleagues that pain is a syndrome in its own right that merits special attention, research, and funding. The arrival of the gate control theory encouraged [him] *to pursue his cause* [and to promote] *the gate control theory as a focus for new medical approaches'.*[14]

The gate control theory offered a plausible explanation for many of the complex neurological findings and therapeutic responses. It produced a rationale for the therapeutic effectiveness of transcutaneous electrical nerve stimulation (TENS), for spinal cord stimulation and for acupuncture, by postulating that these methods could activate afferent (ascending) inhibitory neurons. Antidepressants, biofeedback and a variety of effective cognitive therapies could now be attributed to modulation of central inhibitory neurons in the brain or brainstem.

Beecher and Bonica each developed their concerns for pain during wartime, albeit under very different circumstances. Their work complemented each other's, however, in that each was based on the variability and unpredictability of pain. But remarkably, although Bonica and Beecher were active during exactly the same years and must have been well known to each other, there is no evidence that there was any professional contact between them, nor did they cite each other's work. Nevertheless, working independently, each provided important clues that led to the formulation of the gate control theory, which in turn provided a rationale for the modern treatment of pain.

Treatment and prevention of acute postoperative pain

There are many different causes of chronic pain, in addition to malignant disease, so it is perhaps not surprising that efforts to relieve chronic pain have been only moderately successful. Acute pain, however, is usually associated with some clearly defined lesion, so one might expect that treatment would be more effective. Unfortunately, the availability of effective therapy has not guaranteed that it would be applied appropriately.

The principles had been well established by Beecher and others. Beecher had shown that while most severely wounded soldiers do not complain, most hospital patients complain bitterly following major surgery. Following Beecher's return to civilian practice, he and his associates documented the unsatisfactory state of postoperative pain relief and carried out a programme of research into the appropriate use of analgesic drugs following surgery.

Describing the unsatisfactory medication practices in the early postwar years, Beecher's colleague Arthur Keats wrote that '*Some nurses have been taught that every postoperative patient must have two doses of narcotics during the first postoperative night ... some nurses routinely give all postoperative patients a narcotic at 11:00 p.m. to guarantee a quiet night and time for their other duties*'.[15] Beecher and Keats then attempted to estimate the magnitude of these abuses by comparing the amount of morphine needed with the amount actually received. To estimate need, they allowed patients following cholecystectomy to receive 10 mg of morphine (the standard dose at that time) as often as every hour to control their pain. The hospital records of identical groups of ward (charity), semiprivate and private patients and the amounts of postoperative morphine they received were then tabulated. The ward patients who were allowed to receive morphine on demand as often as hourly were found to have received, on average, 3.2 doses. From the hospital records of ward patients receiving routine pain management, it was found that they had received on average 5.6 doses, semiprivate patients had received 9.8 doses and private patients 13.4. Commenting on this extraordinary finding of medication abuse, Keats wrote that '*with a better understanding of the postoperative patient, it is hoped that an improved treatment of this common and neglected painful state will result'.[15]*

At that time, some patients must have received pain medication in excess of need, but it was more common for postoperative pain to be treated inadequately or inappropriately. Blame for this state of affairs must be apportioned partly to the doctors who wrote inappropriate orders, and partly to the nursing staff who implemented the orders. Patients vary greatly in their perception of postoperative pain and in their need and demand for medication. Needs were not met when medication was given in set doses at set intervals, nor were they met when medication was given 'in minimal doses at the longest intervals because doctors and nurses misunderstood the dangers of overdosage and were afraid of the patients becoming addicted'.

The answer to this problem has been to develop methods by which patients themselves control the frequency and dosage of analgesics. The new technology of 'patient-controlled analgesia' was introduced into clinical practice in the late 1970s and has rapidly become the standard of care in most (though not all) hospitals.[16,17] Small doses of pain-relieving drugs – usually morphine or related opioids – can now be administered by a pump that is activated by a pushbutton held by the patient. The device incorporates various safety controls that ensure that the previous dose has had time to act before the machine will respond to the next demand, and the control device can also be adjusted to set appropriate maximum dosage rates. In addition, there are alarms to alert the nursing staff in case of malfunction. The patient can thus relieve pain when it occurs, but can also anticipate and prevent pain by administering a dose prior to undertaking a painful manoeuvre. While patient-controlled devices have been used for the administration of analgesics by the subcutaneous or intramuscular routes, they have been most successful when used with intravenous or epidural infusions. The introduction of patient-controlled analgesia has transformed the care of patients in the postoperative period.

In recent years, anaesthetists have increasingly used epidural, spinal or other regional local anaesthetic nerve blocks to abolish pain after operations. Usually, a long-acting local anaesthetic is injected at the end of the operation so that the patient has a pain-free period before transferring to intramuscular or oral analgesic drugs. When a continuous epidural anaesthetic is considered more appropriate, the catheter is inserted at the beginning of the operation and the nerve block is maintained during and after the operation by repeated doses or a continuous infusion of the local anaesthetic drug. This technique not only reduces the quantity of general anaesthetic required, but tends to reduce bleeding and minimize circulatory responses to the surgery.

It has now been shown that this so-called 'neuraxial' anaesthesia that interrupts the afferent pain pathways going to the spinal cord and brain during surgery has other advantages. It is believed that the combination of neuraxial anaesthesia with general anaesthesia is associated with a more rapid postoperative recovery, less postoperative pain, and decreased analgesic requirements in the postoperative period. Thus, neuraxial anaesthesia not only protects against the pain of surgical trauma, but can also protect against some of the manifestations of surgical stress. There are, inevitably, some complications associated with the techniques used for neuraxial blockade, so further work will undoubtedly be required to establish the risk/benefit ratio of these exciting developments.

References

1. Bonica J. *The Management of Pain*. Philadelphia: Lea and Febiger, 1953.
2. Pernick MS. *A Calculus of Suffering: Pain, Professionalism, and Anesthesia in Nineteenth Century America*. New York: Columbia University Press, 1985.
3. Ray P. *The History of Pain* (transl by Wallace LE, Cadden JA, Cadden SW). Cambridge, MA: Harvard University Press, 1993.
4. Leriche R. *La chirugie de la douleur*. Paris: Masson, 1937 [Cited in reference 3 above].
5. Jewsbury ECO. Insensitivity to pain. *Brain* 1951;**74**:336–53.
6. Guthrie GJA. *Treatise on Gunshot Wounds*. London: Burgess and Hill, 1827 [Cited in reference 9 below].
7. Dupuytren G, quoted by Lescelliere-Lafusse CC. *Histoire de la cicatrisation de ses modes de formation, et des considérations pathologiques et thérapeutiques qui en découlent*. Montpellier, 1836.
8. Porter JB. Medical and surgical notes of campaigns in the War with Mexico. *American Journal of Medical Sciences* 1852;**23**:33 and 1852;**24**:20.
9. Beecher HK. Relationship of significance of wound to pain experience. *Journal of the American Medical Association* 1956;**161**:1609–13.
10. Marshall HR. *Pain, Pleasure and Aesthetics*. London: Macmillan, 1894 [Cited in reference 9 above].
11. Mitchell SW. *Injuries of Nerves and their Consequences*. Philadelphia: JB Lippincott, 1872.
12. Bonica JJ. Evolution and current status of pain programs. *Journal of Pain Symptom Management* 1990;**5**:368–74.
13. Melzack R, Wall PD. Pain mechanisms: a new theory. *Science* 1965;**150**:971–9.
14. Melzack R. From the gate to the neuromatrix. *Pain* 1999; **Suppl 6**: S121–6.
15. Keats A. Postoperative pain: research and treatment. *Journal of Chronic Diseases* 1956;**4**:72–83.

16. White PF. Use of patient-controlled analgesia for management of acute pain. *Journal of the American Medical Association* 1988;**259**:243–7.
17. Graves DA, Foster TS, Batenhorst RL et al. Patient-controlled analgesia. *Annals of Internal Medicine* 1983;**99**:360–5.

8 Curare: the Indian arrow poison

It was the 16th century explorers who first encountered the deadly poisoned arrows used by the South American Indians, but it was the French scientist La Condamine who traversed the Amazon from the Andes to the sea and bought samples of the poison back to Europe in 1743. Its mysterious properties fascinated scientists for nearly a century before a veterinary surgeon used it to treat tetanus in a horse, but another century was to elapse before it was introduced into anaesthesia.

On the 23 January 1942, a Canadian anaesthetist, Harold Griffith, gave an intravenous injection of a drug called Intocostrin to a powerfully built young man who was having his appendix removed under light anaesthesia with the gas cyclopropane. The result was dramatic. In less than a minute, the tight abdominal muscles relaxed completely and the surgeon was able to insert his hand into the abdomen and remove the appendix with great ease. Over the next few weeks, Griffith and his colleague, Enid Johnson, administered the drug to a further 24 patients with equally good results. The introduction to the paper describing the trial was simple and to the point:

'Every anesthetist has wished at times that he might be able to produce rapid and complete muscular relaxation in resistant patients under general anesthesia. This is a preliminary report on the clinical use of a drug which will give this kind of relaxation, temporarily and apparently quite harmlessly'.[1]

The drug Intocostrin was, in fact, a purified preparation of curare,* one of the deadly arrow poisons that were used by South American Indians

---

* Laurence Keymis, Sir Walter Raleigh's lieutenant, was the first writer to give a name to the poison in 1596. He called it 'ourari'. It is not clear how the name 'curare' came into use, but it is suggested that it arises from European attempts to provide a phonetic equivalent of the local name for the poison, which is variously transcribed as 'urari', 'wourali', 'woorara', etc.

living in the region of the Orinoco, Essequibo and Amazon river basins. We have already noted how the introduction of the intravenous anaesthetic drug thiopental and the muscle relaxant curare revolutionized general anaesthesia. The new technique enabled the patient to be anaesthetized quickly, and, since it avoided the dangers and side-effects of deep anaesthesia (such as circulatory depression), surgeons could begin to operate on higher-risk patients. Furthermore, when anaesthesia was maintained with nitrous oxide as opposed to ether, there was no risk of explosion, so that diathermy could be used to seal bleeding vessels. But what impressed patients most was that induction of anaesthesia was pleasant, that they were awake shortly after the end of surgery, and that they were much less likely to suffer nausea and vomiting after operation. It was, indeed, a major breakthrough. What, then, was curare, and how did it come to be introduced into anaesthesia?

Early reports of the arrow poison

Arrow poisons had been used by many primitive communities since prehistoric times. Some acted on the heart, some produced convulsions, while others caused inflammation, but it was only in South America that the paralysing poison 'curare' or 'woorari' was found (Figure 8.1). Curare was an extremely potent poison derived from a climbing plant in the Amazonian jungle. The preparation of the poison was performed in

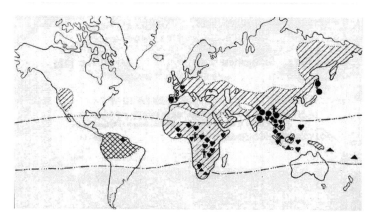

Figure 8.1 Map showing areas where arrow poisons have been used. Paralysing poisons have only been used in Borneo and South America (cross-hatched area). (From Arrow Poisons. Ed. George Rosen. *CIBA Symposia* 1941;**3(7)**:994. Reproduced with permission from John Wiley & Sons Limited.)

secret by certain Indian tribes, who then supplied their neighbours. The poison looked like pitch and was smeared on the tips of small arrows that were fired from a bow or blowpipe – hence the later name for the poison 'the flying death' (Figures 8.2 and 8.3). The tip of the arrow broke off when the arrow hit the prey, and the poison then entered the bloodstream,

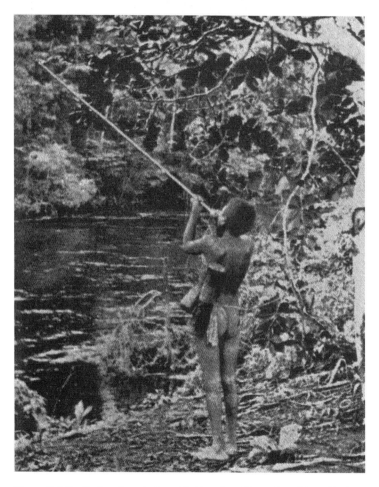

Figure 8.2 South American Indian with blowpipe. (Reproduced from Davison MHA. *The Evolution of Anaesthesia*. Altrincham, UK: John Sherratt and Son, 1965.)

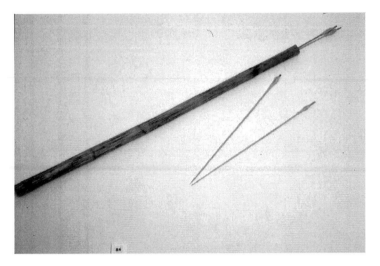

Figure 8.3 Arrows and a section of a blowpipe used by South American Indians to catch their prey. The cotton wound round the blunt end provides a seal with the blowpipe. These were purchased by Keith Sykes from Indians on the Brazilian–Venezuelan border. (Nuffield Department of Anaesthetics, Oxford.)

circulated round the body and paralysed all the skeletal muscles. The prey fell to the ground, and death followed within minutes from respiratory failure and asphyxia.[2]

The first description of the use of poisoned arrows by South American Indians was contained in a collection of letters entitled *De Orbe Novo*, published in 1516.[3] The letters were written by Peter D'Anghera, an Italian church dignitary attached to the court of Isabella of Spain. They were addressed to his friend Ascorio Sforza in Rome, and were based on conversations with explorers who had returned from the newly discovered continent. There are references to poisoned arrows throughout the text. This is from the first 'Decade' of *De Orbe Novo*:

'Two days passed at Santa Cruz, where thirty of our Spaniards placed in an ambuscade saw, from the place where they were watching, a canoe in the distance coming towards them, in which were eight men and as many women. At a given signal they fell upon the canoe; as they approached, the men and women let forth a volley of arrows with great rapidity and accuracy. Before the Spaniards had time to protect themselves with their shields,

one of our men, a Galician, was killed by a woman, and another was seriously wounded by an arrow shot by that same woman. It was discovered that their poisoned arrows contained a kind of liquid which oozed out when the point broke'.[3]

In folio 60 of Richard Eden's 1555 translation of *De Orbe Novo*, we read that:

'this (Indian) kinge layde wayte for oure men. For, as they were filling theire barelles, he set upon them with about seven hundred men . . . armed after theire manner, although they were naked. For only the kinge and his noblemen were appareled . . so fiercely assaylynge oure men with theire venomous arrows that they slewe of them fortie and seven . . . for that poison is of such force, that albeit the woundes were not great, yet they died thereof immediately'.[3]

Antonio de Herrera, who was the official chronicler for Philip II and Philip III of Spain, also mentioned poisoned arrows.[4] He described the extraordinary journey of Francisco de Orellana down the river Amazon. A party of explorers under the command of Gonzalo Pizzaro set out from Quito on Christmas Day 1539, and, after suffering intense cold and other hardships as they crossed the Andes, they eventually reached the upper Amazon basin. Finding their way blocked by forests, they built a ship. Francisco was ordered to descend the river to find food and then return to the main party. He journeyed for some 80 leagues (over 200 miles), but was attacked by male and female natives with poisoned arrows, so he built bulwarks round the ship for protection. He found no food, and did not return to the main party. It is not known whether he was unable to do so because of the strength of the current or whether he deliberately deserted, but he continued down the river and became the first person to complete a voyage down the Amazon from the Andes to its mouth.

Sir Walter Raleigh also mentioned the use of poisoned arrows in his book *The Discoverie of the Large, Rich and Bewtiful Empire of Guiana,* published in 1596, but his descriptions of the mode of death of the victims suggest that they died a lingering death from wound infection. This is quite different from the later descriptions of rapid death from curare.

De la Condamine, and the shape of the Earth

The division of South America between the Spanish and the Portuguese agreed at the Convention of Tordesillas in 1494 virtually closed the continent to explorers from other countries for the next 250 years. Although there are many references to the lethal effects of the poisoned arrows in the Spanish literature during this period, it was Charles Marie de la Condamine, a French naturalist, mathematician and member of L'Académie Royale des Sciences, who brought news of curare to the rest of Europe. It was the Academy that obtained special permission for an expedition designed to resolve one of the major controversies of the time.

In the late 17th and early 18th century, there was much discussion about the shape of the Earth. Newton in his *Principia* (published in 1687) reasoned that the Earth must be an oblate spheroid (flattened at the poles). His view was supported by the Dutch astronomer Christiaan Huygens. In the opposing camp were two French astronomers, Gian Domenico Cassini and his son Jacques. They had measured arcs of the Earth's surface north and south of Paris and concluded that the Earth was a prolate spheroid (flattened at the Equator). To resolve the dispute, the French Academy dispatched two expeditions to measure the distance on the surface of the Earth subtended by an angle of 1°: firstly along a meridian close to the Equator, and secondly along a meridian near to the North Pole. La Condamine and Pierre Bouguer were sent as joint leaders of the expedition to Peru in 1735, while Pierre-Louis Moreau de Maupurtuis led an expedition to Lapland in 1736.

La Condamine spent some eight years making his measurements, and, although the results differed somewhat from those made by Bouguer, they finally confirmed the Newtonian theory. But while he was in Peru, La Condamine also made a number of expeditions into the jungle. He watched the Ticunas Indians making the arrow poison from the roots of creepers and other plants, and he described how they fired the poisoned arrows from bows or through long blowguns. He noted that the animals died quickly after they were hit, and that the Indians appeared to suffer no harm when they ate the animal. Intrigued by the properties of the poison, he injected it into a hen and concluded that the rapid death was caused by paralysis of the respiratory muscles. He then ate the hen without suffering any ill effects, and noted that the flesh was more tender than usual, and that it had an excellent flavour.

In 1743, La Condamine left Quito and spent four months travelling by raft down the Amazon from the Andes to the South Atlantic, mapping the various tributaries of the river as he went.[5] Amazingly, he also confirmed that there was a connection between the Amazon and Orinoco rivers. He wrapped his precious instruments in 'caoutchouc' (the raw rubber obtained from rubber trees) and so became one of the first to use this substance. He brought samples of the arrow poison back to Europe and demonstrated its poisonous properties to scientists in the University of Leyden, then one of the most famous medical schools in Europe.

Early investigations into the mode of action of curare

The remarkable properties of the arrow poison aroused great interest in the scientific community, and la Condamine's samples were soon subjected to further investigation. The next person to study the poison was an English physician, Richard Brocklesbury, who qualified at Leyden in 1745, and subsequently attended Dr Samuel Johnson in his last illness. He may have been present when la Condamine demonstrated the actions of the poison in Leyden. In 1747, Brocklesbury described how the application of the poison to a wound in a cat produced respiratory paralysis, but he also made the important observation that the heart continued to beat for some time after respiration had stopped.[6]

The next investigator to use la Condamine's samples was a French scientist, Monsieur Herissant. He was a Fellow of the Royal Society and sent a communication that was translated into English by Thomas Slack and published in the *Philosophical Transactions* in 1751/52.[7] After describing how he narrowly escaped death from the poison on two occasions,* he proceeded to undertake a series of macabre experiments not only on dogs, rabbits, cats, horses, moles, pigs, rats, mice and young wolves, but also on a bear and an eagle. In one series of experiments, he injected the poison into the extremity of a limb and found that if he cut off the limb immediately, or applied a red-hot iron to the wound, the animal showed no signs of being affected by the poison. This demonstrated that the poison was only effective if it entered the blood stream and circulated round the body.

In 1769, Edwin Bancroft, an English physician, naturalist and explorer, who had spent five years in South America, listed the ingredients used to make the poison, but concluded that the proportions of each ingredient varied from tribe to tribe.[8] He described how the Accawau Indians in Guiana heated the bark from the roots of the various plants in water and

* His paper starts by describing two events which *'had like to have disabled me from prosecuting the work I had undertaken; having narrowly escaped death'*. He then recounts how his young assistant had failed to reappear from the closet where he had been boiling the poison in order to make it more concentrated, and how he had found the boy almost unconscious. He was somewhat put out by this happening, but decided to try a traditional remedy and gave the boy a pint of good wine mixed with sugar. He records that the boy went home *'very merry and happy'*. On the next day, Herissant sat in the closet with the boiling poison himself. Within an hour, he also felt faint. When he tried to leave the closet, he found that he was so weak that he was only just able to drag himself into the yard. However, he too was revived by a large bowl of wine and sugar! His second brush with death resulted from the explosion of one of the glass phials into which he had put the poison. This shattered on a hot day when he was not wearing a shirt and produced a number of cuts on his chest, but apparently none of the poison entered the bloodstream, for he noted no ill effect.

how the Indians then extracted the poison by squeezing the bark with their bare hands, noting that they took good care not to have any broken skin when they did so. He also described the small arrows used with the blowpipe. These were about 30 cm long and 3–4 mm in diameter.* The poison, which looked like pitch, was applied to the point of the arrow and a small quantity of cotton was wound round the rear end to make an airtight connection with the smooth interior of the blowgun. The latter was about 3–4 metres long and fashioned from a type of bamboo (Figure 8.3).

Another person who studied the poison was the Abbé Felix Fontana in Florence.[9] He was an experimental scientist and the Director of the Cabinet of Natural History of the Grand Duke of Tuscany. He had been working for two years on the mode of action of snake venom and had performed some 4000 experiments on 600 viper snakes. In 1780, he travelled to London to obtain samples of the curare poison from the celebrated English physician Dr William Heberden. Fontana had previously made important observations on nerves and muscles, and carried out a series of carefully planned experiments with curare. He showed that the poison produced no effect if he applied it directly to an exposed nerve in a rabbit. This caused him to conclude that curare exerted its effect by a direct action on the muscles. He noted that the poison did not affect the heart muscle, and he also showed that if he prevented the curare from entering the circulation by applying a tourniquet proximal to the site of injection, the animal survived.

Next on the scene was the English surgeon Benjamin Brodie, who was also interested in poisons. In 1811–12 he conducted a number of studies on the effects of various poisons on the body, and began to experiment with some of the samples of curare that had been brought back to England by Edwin Bancroft.[10] These samples were provided by Bancroft's son, Edward Nathaniel Bancroft, a physician to St George's Hospital, London, and he assisted Brodie with the experiments. Brodie confirmed Brocklesbury's observation that the heart continued to beat after respiration had ceased, but he took the experiment one stage further and showed that that he could keep the animal alive by intermittently forcing air into the lungs with a bellows. This provided the key to the future clinical use of the drug. As Brodie wrote:

'Having learned that the circulation might be kept up by artificial respiration for a considerable time after the woorara had produced its full effects, it occurred to me, that in an animal under the influence of this or any other poison that acts in a

* Waterton brought some of these arrows back to England. They may be viewed, together with other Waterton artefacts, in the museum in Wakefield, Yorkshire.

> *similar manner, by continuing the artificial respiration for a*
> *sufficient length of time after natural respiration had ceased, the*
> *brain might recover from the impression which the poison had*
> *produced, so that it would be restored to life.'*

He subsequently tested this theory in a cat. After 40 minutes of artificial respiration, the cat suddenly wakened and walked away. Brodie also found that if he injected the curare into a limb distal to a tourniquet, the curare had no effect until the tourniquet was released, so confirming Herissant's and Fontana's earlier observations that the poison only worked when it entered the blood stream.[11]

Charles Waterton, the squire of Walton Hall

The most colourful character in the history of curare was Charles Waterton, a Yorkshireman who moved to British Guiana in 1804 to manage his family's plantation (Figure 8.4). He was one of the great

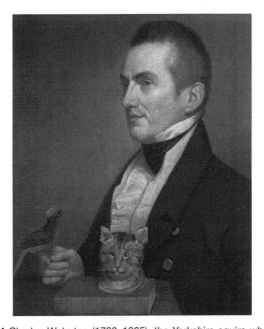

Figure 8.4 Charles Waterton (1782–1865), the Yorkshire squire who made a number of expeditions into the Amazon rain forest and brought specimens of curare back to England. (Painting by Charles Wilson Peale, 1824. Reproduced with permission from the National Portrait Gallery, London.)

eccentrics of his time. He was a devout Catholic and could not understand why the Pope would not receive him after he and a friend had scaled the dome of St Peter's in Rome. They had hung their gloves on the top of the lightning conductor, and then stood on the head of the statue of an angel on the Castel Sant' Angelo. Waterton was a fearless naturalist who fought large snakes with his bare hands and rode on the back of a small crocodile before killing it and stuffing it. He was also one of the first persons to create a bird sanctuary on his Yorkshire estate.[12]

Between 1812 and 1824, Waterton undertook a series of expeditions into the South American jungle (Figure 8.5). These resulted in his fascinating book *Wanderings in South America*,[13] first published in 1825.* In this book, he gave detailed descriptions of how the natives used either poisoned darts fired from a long blow-pipe, poisoned arrows, or poisoned spears to catch their prey, and he noted that they could kill an animal at a range of 100 metres when using the blowpipe. Waterton communicated these results to Sir Joseph Banks (the British explorer and naturalist who had sailed round the world with Captain James Cook in 1768–69, and who had become a long-term President of the Royal Society), and Banks queried whether the poison would be effective against large animals. On his return to Guiana, Waterton tested the poison on dogs, an ox and a sloth, and demonstrated that, if the dose was increased appropriately, quite large animals could be killed by the poison. Waterton was present when Brodie and a veterinary surgeon named William Sewell repeated the artificial ventilation experiment on a donkey at the Veterinary College in London in 1814, although Waterton did not mention Brodie's part in the procedure. Here is Waterton's description of the experiment:

---

* Waterton's escapades make fascinating reading. He was in the habit of bleeding himself regularly in the belief that this would maintain his health. He describes how he once journeyed with a Scottish gentleman called Tarbet. They both slept in their hammocks in the thatched loft of a planter's house, but the Scotsman was severely bitten by vampire bats whilst Waterton was not touched. He records that when he woke up he had put his colleague into a worse humour by remarking that '*an European surgeon would not have been so generous as to have blooded him without making a charge*'. Waterton also describes how he had deliberately left his foot exposed all night on many occasions but was most disappointed to find that vampires never bit him. The poor Scotsman suffered even more on a later occasion when he had a severe gastrointestinal upset after eating some crabs. Waterton decorates his delicate description of the events with a number of highly appropriate Latin quotations, but the gist of the story is that during one of his nocturnal trips to the outside loo, the Scotsman sat down on the seat only to discover that it was unfortunately in the path of the annual migration of a particularly vicious species of ant. As Waterton commented, '*had he dropped a lighted match on a pound of gunpowder, it could not have caused a greater recoil*'!

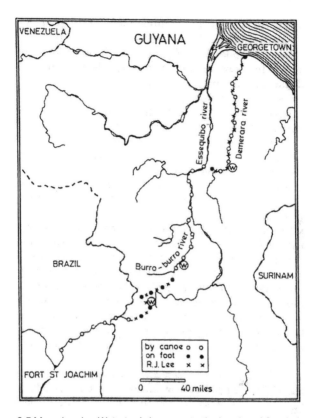

Figure 8.5 Map showing Waterton's journeys to the interior of South America. (From Smith WDA. Proceedings of a Symposium Held to Commemorate the Bicentenary of Charles Waterton (1782–1865). Waterton and Wourali. *British Journal of Anaesthesia* 1983;**55**:221–33. © The Board and Management and Trustees of the *British Journal of Anaesthesia*. Reproduced by permission of Oxford University Press/*British Journal of Anaesthesia*.)

> 'A she-ass received the wourali poison in the shoulder, and died apparently in 10 minutes. An incision was made in its windpipe, and through it the lungs were regularly inflated for two hours with a pair of bellows. Suspended animation returned. The ass held up her head and looked around; but the inflating being discontinued, she sunk once more in apparent death. The artificial breathing was immediately recommenced, and continued without intermission for two hours more. This saved

the ass from final dissolution; she rose up, and walked about; she seemed neither in agitation nor in pain. The wound, through which the poison entered, was healed without difficulty. Her constitution, however, was so severely affected, that it was long a doubt if ever she would be well again. She looked lean and sickly for above a year, but began to mend the spring after; and by Midsummer became fat and frisky'. He added *'The kind hearted reader will rejoice on learning that Earl Percy, pitying her misfortunes, sent her down from London to Walton Hall, near Wakefield).* There she goes by the name Wouralia. Wouralia shall be sheltered from the wintry storm; and when the summer comes she shall feed in the finest pasture. No burden shall be placed on her and she shall end her days in peace'.* In later editions he added as a footnote to the original description: *'Poor Wouralia breathed her last on the 15th of February 1839, having survived the operation nearly five and twenty years'.*[4]

She also received an obituary in the local newspaper.

Mechanism of action

By the mid-19th century, physiology was becoming an established science, and in 1842, the French physiologist and founder of experimental medicine, Claude Bernard, conducted a series of experiments on the mechanism of action of the poison in the laboratory of M Pelouze (Figure 8.6). He had become interested in the drug because he had been a student of François Magendie, a French physiologist who contributed fundamental knowledge about the function of the nervous system. Before 1846, there were no anaesthetics, so Magendie used curare to keep animals still during his experiments. Unfortunately, this practice continued until the end of the century in some laboratories, and ultimately led to the creation of the Royal Commission on Vivisection in 1875.

Bernard was curious to know how curare exerted its effect, and conducted a series of experiments in frogs. He showed that, even when the animal was totally paralysed, electrical impulses were still passing along the nerves. Since the muscles continued to respond to direct electrical stimulation, he concluded that the drug must block the conduction of the nerve impulse from the nerve to the muscle fibres. These remarkable observations were published in 1850–57, but Bernard continued to publish reports of further experiments over the ensuing 30

---

* This was Waterton's home. Waterton's taxidermy specimens, poisoned arrows and other memorabilia are in the nearby museum in Wakefield, Yorkshire.

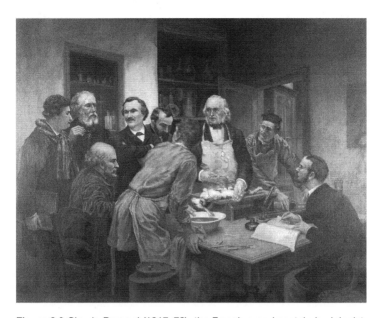

Figure 8.6 Claude Bernard (1817–78), the French experimental physiologist, with some of his pupils in the laboratories. He concluded that curare must act at some point between the nerve and the muscle – the site we now know as the neuromuscular junction. (Reproduced with permission from the Wellcome Library for the History and Understanding of Medicine, London.)

years.[14] These were summarized in his book *La Science Expérimentale* that was published in 1878 (Figure 8.7).

It was not until the mid-1930s, however, that Sir Henry Dale and other scientists showed how the transmission of the electrical nerve impulse to the muscle is effected by the release of tiny packages of the chemical transmitter acetylcholine at the nerve endings. The nerve endings are situated close to a specialized area of muscle (the muscle endplate). This contains receptors that respond to the acetylcholine and trigger an electrical contraction of the muscle fibre. The acetylcholine is immediately destroyed by the enzyme cholinesterase so that the muscle is ready to respond to further nerve impulses. These processes follow each other in rapid succession and so sustain contraction of the muscle, the strength of the contraction being directly related to the frequency of the nerve impulses. Curare acts by occupying a proportion of the receptors,

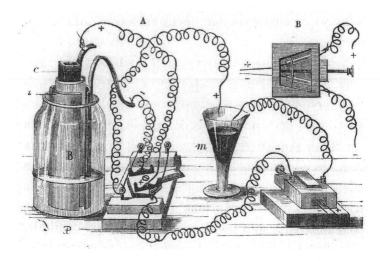

Figure 8.7 Apparatus for electrical stimulation of a nerve used by Claude Bernard to establish the site of action of curare. (Reproduced with permission from the Wellcome Library for the History and Understanding of Medicine, London.)

thus blocking the action of acetylcholine. The antagonist to curare, neostigmine, acts by antagonizing the action of the cholinesterase.

The problem of how curare and similar drugs block the neuromuscular junction has stimulated many distinguished scientists to enter this field of research. As a result, we now have a detailed knowledge of how the electrical impulse is conducted down the nerve, and how this impulse causes the muscle to contract. We know how certain drugs stimulate receptors and how other drugs block receptors, and we have reached such a degree of sophistication in drug development that we can tailor the molecular configuration of a drug so that it fits a given receptor anywhere in the body. We understand how the transmission of the nerve impulse to the muscle may be affected by alterations in electrolyte balance and the acid–base status of the blood, and we know more about the way in which the neuromuscular junction is affected by poisons such as botulinum toxin (the popular Botox injection that smoothes the wrinkles of the not-so-young) or by diseases such as myasthenia gravis. Many of these discoveries were stimulated by the interest in curare.

The interest in the unique properties of curare naturally led clinicians to attempt to use it in clinical practice. As early as 1812, William Sewell, the veterinarian who took part in the experiments on the ass with Brodie and Waterton, had suggested that curare might be of use in controlling the muscle spasms in patients who were suffering from rabies and tetanus. As we shall see, 140 years were to pass before his suggestion was successfully implemented.

References

1. Griffith HR, Johnson GE. The use of curare in general anesthesia. *Anesthesiology* 1942;**3**:418–20.
2. Burnap TK, Little DM, eds. *The Flying Death. Classic Papers and Commentary on Curare. (International Anesthesiology Clinics*, Vol 6, Part 2). Boston: Little, Brown, 1968.
3. MacNutt FA, ed. *De Orbe Novo. The Eight Decades of Peter Martyr D'Anghera. Translated from the Latin with Notes and Introduction*, Vols 1 and 2. New York: Lennox Hill (Burt Franklin), Reprinted 1970.
4. McIntyre AR. *Curare. Its History, Nature and Clinical Use*. Chicago: University of Chicago Press, 1947.
5. De La Condamine M. Relation abrégée d'un Voyage fait dans l'intérieur de l'Amérique méridionale, depuis la Côte de la Mer du Sud jusques aux Côtes du Brésil et de la Guiane, en descendant la riviére des Amazones. *Histoire de l'academie Royale des Sciences* 1745: 391–492.
6. Brocklesby RA. Letter to the President of the Royal Society concerning the Indian poison, sent over from M. de la Condamine. *Philosophical Transactions of the Royal Society of London* 1747;**44(ii)**:407–12.
7. Herissant M. Experiments made on a great number of living animals, with the poison of Lamas, and of Ticunas. Translated from the French by Tho. Stack. *Philosophical Transactions of the Royal Society of London* 1751/52;**47**:75–92.
8. Bancroft E. An essay on the natural history of Guiana and South America. London: T Becket and PA De Hont, 1769.
9. Fontana F. An essay on the American poison called Ticunas. *Philosophical Transactions of the Royal Society of London* 1780;**70(i)**:163–220 (English translation: Appendix, 9–45).
10. Brodie BC. Experiments and observations on the different modes in which death is produced by certain vegetable poisons. *Philosophical Transactions of the Royal Society of London* 1811;**101**:178–208.
11. Brodie BC. Further experiments and observations on the actions of poisons on the animal system. *Philosophical Transactions of the Royal Society of London* 1812;**102**:205–227.
12. Blackburn J. *Charles Waterton 1782–1865. Traveller and Conservationist*. London: Vintage, 1997.
13. Waterton C. *Wanderings in South America*. London: MacMillan, 1825 (reprinted 1879).
14. Bernard C. On the effects of toxic and medicinal substances. 1857 (translated from the French). In: Faulconer A, Keys TE, eds. *Foundations of Anesthesiology*, Vol 2. Springfield, IL: Charles C Thomas, 1965: 1142–50.

Further reading

Smith P. *Arrows of Mercy*. Garden City, NY: Doubleday, 1969.

Sykes WS. *Essays on the First 100 Years of Anaesthesia*, Vol 1. Edinburgh: E & S Livingstone, 1960: 86–98.

Thomas KB. *Curare. Its History and Usage*. Philadelphia: JB Lippincott, 1963.

9 Spasms and convulsions: the role of curare

Spasms and convulsions occur in diseases such as epilepsy, tetanus (lockjaw) and rabies (hydrophobia). They are frightening and often fatal, so it is not surprising that physicians should have tried to reduce the intensity of spasms by administering curare. In practice, the drug proved to be potentially as lethal as the disease itself: it was only when anaesthetic techniques for supporting ventilation were introduced in the 1950s that lives were saved.

Early attempts to use curare in veterinary and medical practice

Although little was known about the chemistry and pharmacology of curare, this did not deter clinicians from attempting to use the crude preparation therapeutically. It was William Sewell, the veterinary surgeon who had been present when Brodie and Waterton gave curare to the ass Wouralia in 1814 (see Chapter 8), who was the first to use the poison in the treatment of tetanus in animals.[1] Since this disease produces severe muscle stiffness accompanied by intermittent muscle spasms, Sewell reasoned that if he gave curare to paralyse the muscles and then provided artificial ventilation with a bellows connected to the trachea, he might be able to keep the animal alive while the disease burnt itself out. He tried this treatment on two horses with tetanus in 1838. As Sewell wrote later, *'to effect restoration from suspended animation requires about four hours of artificial respiration, to be kept up with great regularity. Neither of the animals on which I tried it died from the experiment or the return of the tetanus; one died from inanition, and the other from repletion'.*[2] Veterinary surgeons were the equal of physicians when they needed to safeguard their reputation by obfuscation.

Another person who was interested in the drug was Francis Sibson, the Resident Apothecary and Surgeon at Nottingham General Infirmary. In 1838, he wrote to Waterton suggesting that curare might be used to treat the convulsions that occurred in patients with rabies. Waterton visited Sibson and watched him give curare to an ass and keep it alive by ventilating the lungs with a bellows. As Waterton recorded, the ass was kept alive for seven hours *'by my worthy friend, Mr Sibson, who exerted himself in a manner that astonished all the company'*. Despite their friendship, Waterton would only agree to provide the curare if he were allowed to be present at the administration. Shortly afterwards, Police Inspector Phelps was bitten on the nose by a rabid dog; unfortunately, he expired before Waterton could reach Nottingham.

Trials in hospital patients

The first recorded administration of curare to a patient with tetanus was by LA Sayre and FA Burrall, surgeon and house-surgeon at Bellevue Hospital, New York, in 1858.[3] Seven days after injuring his hand in a fall from a ladder, an Irish labourer developed classical symptoms of tetanus, with stiffness of the neck and other muscles, followed by severe muscle spasms in the jaws, neck, thorax and abdomen. The spasms of the face muscles produced the characteristic distorted smile known as 'risus sardonicus', while the intense spasms of the back muscles caused the back to be arched backwards to such an extent that the body was supported by the heels and the head – a state known as 'opisthotonos' (Figure 9.1).

The case report describes the distressing effects of the disease, and the even more unpleasant treatment suffered by the patient at that time. Chloroform was given twice for surgical treatment of the hand infection, but each administration precipitated further spasms. The patient was given pain-killing drugs, brandy and beef tea in liberal doses. A blister (counter-irritant) was applied to the spine and attempts were made to administer quinine and brandy, but the patient could not swallow the medicine. It was considered that he was a suitable case for trial of the woorari poison, and a watery solution of this preparation was applied to the wound. He was given a number of enemas (including brandy and beef tea), but these precipitated further spasms. Woorari was applied to the wound on three further occasions, but the patient died during a severe spasm on the day after admission. This is but one example of the bizarre treatment that patients had to endure in those days. Death must have been a merciful release from both the disease and its treatment.

In 1859, the English surgeon Spencer Wells (inventor of the haemostatic forceps still used today) gave curare to three patients who

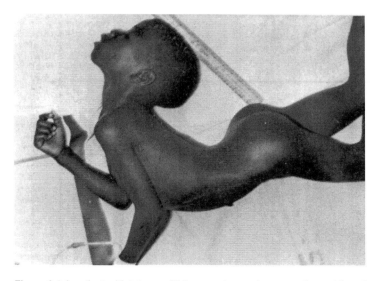

Figure 9.1 A patient with tetanus. All the muscles are in spasm, the arching of the back being caused by contraction of the powerful back muscles. (Reproduced from 1951–1976: Twenty-Five Years of the Faculty of Medicine University of Natal.)

had developed tetanus after gynaecological surgery.[4] Only one patient survived. At about this time, a number of French, German and Italian clinicians, who were influenced by the experimental work being conducted by the physiologist Claude Bernard in France (see Chapter 8), attempted to use curare to reduce the severity of the convulsions in other conditions such as strychnine poisoning, rabies and epilepsy. Few of these patients survived: there was an enormous variation in the potency of the different preparations used for treatment, and it is difficult to produce relaxation of the major skeletal muscles without producing considerable weakness of the muscles of respiration. Since methods of maintaining artificial ventilation for long periods had not yet been developed, patients who received an adequate therapeutic dose of curare usually died from respiratory inadequacy.

Renewed interest

Renewed interest in the therapeutic use of curare was stimulated by Ranyard West, an English physician, who, in 1932, reported that curare could reduce the extreme muscle stiffness seen in some patients with neurological disease.[5] Two years later, Leslie Cole, a physician working at Addenbrooke's Hospital in Cambridge, described the use of subcutaneous injections of curare in the treatment of two patients with tetanus, one of whom survived. Shortly afterwards, West described how he had given an intravenous infusion of curare to 10 patients with tetanus, one of whom had survived. West was still using a crude preparation of curare, and later reported that, in some patients, the drug produced an allergic type of reaction with severe wheezing due to bronchospasm. Because of this problem, West encouraged Harold King, Head of the Chemistry Division of the National Institute for Medical Research, to try to identify the active principle. In 1935, King reported that he had successfully extracted the active component, d-tubocurarine, from a specimen of crude curare obtained from a museum,[6] but although d-tubocurarine became commercially available in 1936, it does not appear to have entered clinical use until Cecil Gray and John Halton began to use it in anaesthesia in Liverpool in 1944.[7]

There is one other prescient study that is of great interest. In 1934, HW Florey, HE Harding and P Fildes from the Department of Pathology at the University of Sheffield, published a paper in *The Lancet* in which they suggested that patients with tetanus could be spared the discomfort of increased muscle tone and spasms by keeping them continuously anaesthetized with a general anaesthetic such as nitrous oxide or ether. They could then be paralysed with repeated doses of curare, while lung ventilation was maintained by nursing them in a Drinker respirator (iron lung). Professor Florey (later famous for his role in the development of penicillin at Oxford) and his colleagues attempted to apply this technique to rabbits that had been infected with tetanus, but the technical difficulties proved to be too great, and the rabbits died.[8] It is of interest that the authors of this paper, who were pathologists and not clinicians, suggested that special units should be set up for applying this type of treatment. Twenty years were to pass before Bjørn Ibsen in Copenhagen successfully treated a patient suffering from tetanus with curare and artificial ventilation, and it was a further 10 years before intensive care units became an integral part of the medical scene.

Richard Gill in Ecuador

The story then moves to Richard C Gill, who has described his lengthy odyssey in his book *White Water: and Black Magic*.[9] Gill was born in the USA in 1901 and expected to follow his father and elder brother into medicine, but after two years of premedical studies at Cornell University, New York, he abandoned the course and went to sea in a tramp steamer. He then spent a year working on a whaling station in the South Georgia Sea. He returned to Cornell, graduated with a degree in English in 1924, and then worked as a schoolteacher and a ranger in Yellowstone National Park. He obtained a job as a salesman for a rubber company in South America in 1928, but left when trade was hit by the 1929 depression. Later, he and his wife Ruth returned to Ecuador and, after eight months of exploration, purchased 750 acres of land at an altitude of about 5000 feet on the eastern slopes of the Andes. Here they built what was probably the first dude ranch in South America.[10] For the next two years, they farmed and led an idyllic life on the edge of the jungle at the Rio Negro ranch (Figure 9.2).

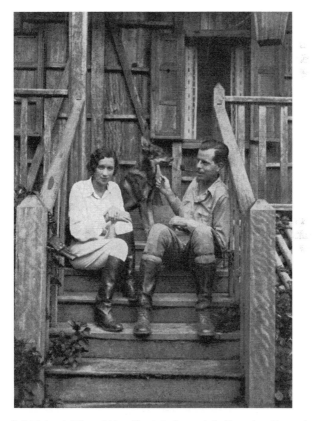

Figure 9.2 Richard Gill and his wife at their ranch in Ecuador. (Reproduced from Gill, RC. Robinson Crusoe in Ecuador. *National Geographic Magazine* 1934; **LXV(2)**; 133–172.)

During this period, Gill made a number of expeditions to the interior and established excellent relationships with several of the Indian tribes. He became very interested in some of their herbal preparations, and persuaded the witch-doctors to allow him to witness the making of the arrow poison (Figure 9.3). He was even granted the status of witch-doctor by the Indians themselves. In 1932, he developed neurological symptoms that were attributed to a fall from a horse, but these were eventually diagnosed as being due to multiple sclerosis. In 1934, when he was severely affected by a paralysis that was accompanied by severe muscle spasms, he and his neurologist, Walter Freeman,* discussed the possibility of using curare to ameliorate the spasms. This reawakened Gill's interest in curare and made him determined to return to the jungle. He devised his own course of intensive physiotherapy, was able to drive a car by 1936, and by 1938 was able to walk with a stick. Meanwhile, he

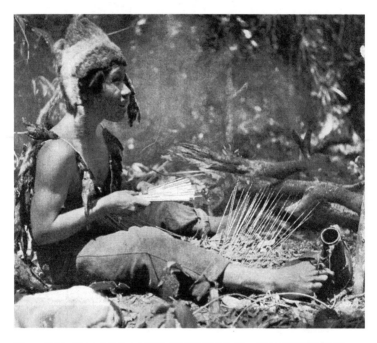

Figure 9.3 Indian preparing poison arrows. (Reproduced from Gill, RC. Robinson Crusoe in Ecuador. *National Geographic Magazine* 1934; **LXV(2)**; 133–172.)

* Freeman was the neurologist who later introduced the operation of prefrontal lobotomy.

was teaching himself botany, and making detailed plans for an expedition to collect more crude curare and other herbal medicines that he believed might help alleviate disease. Luckily, he met a wealthy businessman, Sayre Merrill, who agreed to finance the expedition.

The 1938 expedition

In May 1938, Gill set out from Guayaquil with an expedition that eventually consisted of 4 Ecuadorian assistants, 75 Indian porters and 4 subchiefs, 36 mules and 6 riding animals, 12 canoes and their crews, and 2 tons of equipment.[11] The journey to the jungle campsite selected by Gill took three weeks and involved perilous descents through rapids, ravines and thick jungle. The party spent five months in the jungle and brought back about 75 plant specimens and some 12 kg of crude curare. When he returned to New York, Gill learnt that the pharmaceutical company Merck, which had been supplying a crude preparation of curare to a psychiatrist, Michael S Burman, for therapeutic trials in patients with severe muscle stiffness, had lost interest in the drug. Merck's refusal to purify his large collection of crude curare specimens was a bitter blow.

Use in psychiatric patients

AE Bennett, a psychiatrist practising in Omaha, Nebraska, was also upset by the Merck decision to withdraw the supply. He had read Burman's papers on the muscle relaxation produced by curare and was hoping to test the effectiveness of curare in the prevention of traumatic complications that occurred in patients who were being given convulsive shock therapy to treat depression. At that time, the convulsions were produced by the injection of pentylenetetrazole (Metrazol), a synthetic central nervous system stimulant. Fortunately, Bennett met Walter Freeman, the neurologist who was looking after Gill, and learnt that Gill had returned with further supplies of curare. Bennett then met Gill in May 1939, and Gill agreed to supply him with some of the crude drug.[12]

It so happened that AR McIntyre, Chairman of the Department of Pharmacology of the University of Nebraska College of Medicine, had a research grant from Squibb Laboratories and had also received some of the drug. He agreed to standardize it, and Bennett used this preparation in his early trials. In August 1939, ER Squibb and Son agreed to buy Gill's entire supply of curare, and, later that year, one of their chemists, Horace Holaday, devised the 'rabbit head drop test' to measure the paralysing power of the purified preparation, which he named 'Intocostrin'. Whereas King had extracted *d*-tubocurarine from a museum specimen of curare of unknown botanical origin, in 1943 two Squibb scientists, Oskar

Wintersteiner and James D Dutcher, reported that they had been able to extract an alkaloid similar to *d*-tubocurarine from the bark of a vine indentified as *Chondodendron tomentosum*.[13] This, at last, identified the source of the active principle of the crude preparation. It is of interest that curare has also been shown to be present in the bark of another vine, *Strychnos toxifera*, which is found mainly in the eastern regions – the area investigated by Charles Waterton.

At the time when Bennett introduced curare into psychiatric practice, the therapeutic convulsions produced by the injection of pentylene-tetrazole were associated with a 20% incidence of dislocations and a 40–50% incidence of compressive spinal fractures – a terrible toll for a dubious cure. Although many psychiatrists initially refused to use Intocostrin because they believed that the beneficial effects of the treatment were produced by the convulsion itself, rather than the associated electrical activity in the brain, the use of Intocostrin spread rapidly within the USA. Within a year or two, it was recognized that the use of curare had greatly reduced the incidence of skeletal damage, and the technique was applied in electroconvulsive therapy (ECT) when this superseded pentylenetetrazole as a method of treatment.[11]

There are three surprising aspects of this early use of curare. First, although psychiatrists had not received any special training in artificial respiration, there appear to have been few deaths due to overdose. This was probably due to the use of a standardized preparation given in relatively low dose. It was also recognized that the drug could be antagonized by neostigmine. The second point of interest is that the electric shock was given to the partially curarized, but conscious, patient. The concept of anaesthetizing the patient with thiopental (Pentothal) before giving the shock was not introduced until 1945. Third, although curare was used in a few patients in the UK in 1939, it was not used frequently until the late 1940s.[14]

The successful use of curare to control the spasms during convulsion therapy sparked off two further developments: the use of curare in anaesthesia (the subject of the next chapter) and its use in the treatment of tetanus.

Successful treatment of tetanus

We described earlier how previous attempts to use curare to abolish the extreme muscle stiffness and life-threatening spasms associated with severe tetanus had failed because a dose that was sufficient to abolish the spasms also produced respiratory paralysis. What was needed was a technique of providing adequate artificial ventilation over prolonged periods. This was achieved in 1929 when Philip Drinker and his colleagues in Boston introduced the first practical tank ventilator – popularly known as the 'iron lung'.[15] The patient lay on a mattress in a large iron cylinder, with the head protruding through an airtight rubber seal at one end. A large bellows driven by an electric motor rhythmically lowered the pressure inside the tank, thereby inflating the lungs (Figure 9.4). The lungs deflated when the pressure was returned to atmospheric. This device was cumbersome but effective, and saved the lives of many patients who suffered from respiratory muscle paralysis due to poliomyelitis.

It was this device that was used in 1947 by two physicians, Vernon C Turner and Thomas C Galloway, working at the Northwestern University School of Medicine in Evanston, Illinois.[16] They treated an 18-year-old

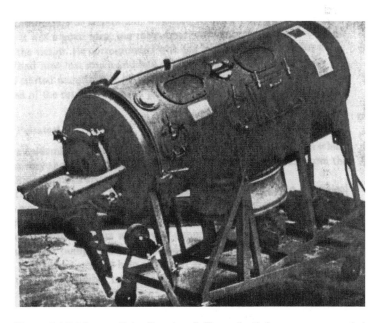

Figure 9.4 Drinker ventilator ('iron lung'). The patient's lungs were expanded by intermittently lowering the pressure inside the tank by means of a large electrically driven bellows. Expiration occurred when the tank pressure was returned to atmospheric pressure. (Reproduced with kind permission from the Association of Anaesthetists of Great Britain and Ireland from Woollam CHM. The development of apparatus for intermittent negative pressure ventilation. *Anaesthesia* 1976;**31**:537–47 and 666–85.)

girl who had developed severe tetanus from an infected wound, and first attempted to use a partial-paralysis regime using *d*-tubocurarine supplemented with doses of Intocostrin. They soon found that a dose of muscle relaxant that suppressed the convulsions also produced respiratory depression, so they decided to perform a tracheostomy to permit removal of secretions, and to use a tank ventilator to provide artificial ventilation. The curare was discontinued after 12 days and the patient survived. In a footnote, the authors gave credit to the members of the Department of Anesthesiology who had administered the curare, aspirated the secretions and supervised the use of the tank ventilator. The cynic might claim that the physicians did the thinking while the anaesthetists did the work.

In 1952, Ronald Woolmer (later Professor in the Research Department of Anaesthetics at the Royal College of Surgeons in London) and JE Cates reported that they had used an intravenous infusion of the newly introduced short-acting muscle relaxant succinylcholine (suxamethonium) to treat severe tetanus in a woman aged 45.[17] They had connected an anaesthetic breathing circuit to the patient's lungs via a tube inserted into the trachea and had maintained ventilation by manually compressing the reservoir bag for several days. In 1954, Lassen and his colleagues in Copenhagen reported that they had successfully treated a 10-year-old girl with severe tetanus using nitrous oxide sedation and intravenous injections of curare. She had required manual ventilation for 18 days, but recovered completely.[18]

It was obvious that few hospitals could provide the staff or facilities to maintain manual artificial ventilation for many days in patients with tetanus, and in 1954 GE Honey and colleagues in Oxford reported the successful use of curare, tracheostomy and mechanical artificial ventilation with the newly developed Radcliffe ventilator (Figure 9.5). This was a mechanical version of the Oxford inflating bellows in which the lungs were inflated by intermittent positive pressure applied to the trachea instead of the intermittent negative pressure around the chest that was employed in the tank ventilator. The authors pointed out that there were dangers in using nitrous oxide for prolonged periods of sedation, and advocated the use of barbiturate drugs for this purpose. They also provided details of the special nursing care and physiotherapy required to ensure a successful outcome; these techniques were gradually adopted by others undertaking this type of care.[19]

Although the technique of intermittent positive-pressure ventilation with a mechanical ventilator was adopted by a few other centres, it was difficult for most general hospitals to provide the necessary staff and facilities. Attempts to treat tetanus cases in small side-wards resulted in

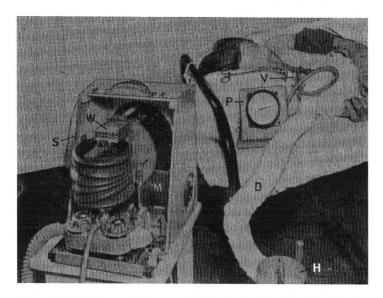

Figure 9.5 Radcliffe respiration pump (left), hot water humidifier (H, right) with lagged pipe (D) leading to inflation valve (V). A lever driven by an electric motor (M) expanded the bellows, which filled with an air/oxygen mixture. The weights on top of the bellows (W) then forced the air into the patient through the inflation valve (V) that was connected to the tracheostomy tube. The inflation pressure was measured with the gauge (P), and the volume of gas leaving the lungs was measured with a gas meter. The respiratory rate was controlled by a four-speed gearbox and manually operated clutch to provide eight respiration rates, and the machine was powered by 230V or 12V electric motors. (Nuffield Department of Anaesthetics, Oxford.)

deaths from accidental disconnection of ventilator tubes, blockage of the tracheostomy tube by dried secretions, or other mishaps. So, for a number of years, satisfactory results were only obtained in a relatively small number of centres that specialized in this type of treatment. It was not until the mid-1960s that intensive care units suitable for treating such cases began to appear in District General Hospitals in the UK.

Use of curare in babies with tetanus

Tetanus is caused by a bacillus that survives in agricultural land fertilized by animal manure, and can enter the body through a wound. African mothers often applied cow dung to the baby's umbilical cord, and this resulted in a severe form of tetanus that was associated with a mortality rate of 80–85%. In August 1959, Pat Smythe, a paediatrician, and Arthur Bull, a paediatric anaesthetist, in Capetown, South Africa reported that they had used curare and mechanical artificial ventilation to treat 10 newborn babies with severe tetanus and that 8 had survived.[20] Earlier in that year, Professor EB Adams had invited the present author (KS) to set up a respiration unit in the Department of Medicine in the King Edward VIII Hospital in Durban, a teaching hospital that catered for the African and Asian population. The aim was to set up a randomized controlled trial to compare the new technique of treating tetanus using curare and mechanical ventilation with the standard sedation regime in adults with severe tetanus. To the Durban doctors' surprise, the usual three or four adult admissions per week suffering from severe tetanus did not materialize, so after three weeks of relative inactivity, it was decided to treat two babies who were suffering from severe neonatal tetanus (Figure 9.6). The three ventilators brought from England were designed for adults, so it was necessary to devise new breathing systems in order that only a small fraction of the gas delivered by the ventilator entered the

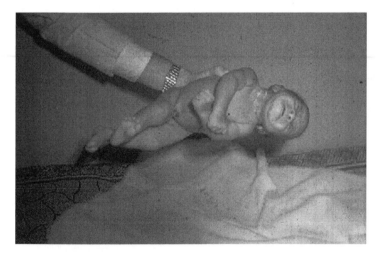

Figure 9.6 Baby with neonatal tetanus showing the rigid body resulting from the increased muscle tone. All the skeletal muscles are contracting continuously, so that respiration is impaired. Respiration stops completely during the intermittent spasms. (Photograph taken in King Edward VIII Hospital, Durban, South Africa by Keith Sykes.)

babies' lungs. We had to devise new tracheostomy tubes and methods of humidifying the inspired gases, and we had to learn how to clear secretions from the lungs and perform the myriad other tasks that are essential for a successful outcome (Figure 9.7). The results of the trial, published by Ralph Wright and colleagues in 1961, revealed a mortality rate of 85% in the group given the traditional treatment with sedation and 44% in the group given curare and mechanical ventilation.[21] The mortality rate with curare was subsequently reduced to 11%.[22] These studies showed conclusively that life could be sustained artificially while the patient was protected from the effects of the muscle spasms by curare (Figure 9.8). They also showed that it was possible to take over a body function (in this case, breathing) and to maintain it artificially for prolonged periods. By the early 1960s, it was realized that the long-term control of ventilation was a practicable proposition and that special units needed to be developed to enable this technique to be applied to tetanus and other conditions requiring ventilatory support. This finally gave the impetus to the development of intensive care units as we know them today.

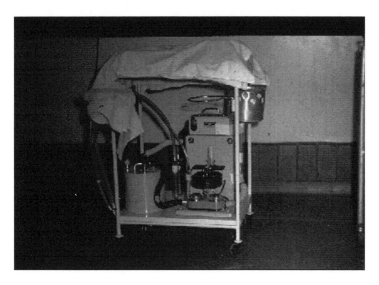

Figure 9.7 Radcliffe ventilator (bottom right) and humidifier (bottom left) in Durban. The large tin can with holes in the side was an improvized bacterial filter for the inspired air. The towel covered sterile suction catheters and replacement tracheal and tracheostomy tubes. (Photograph taken in King Edward VIII Hospital, Durban, South Africa by Keith Sykes.)

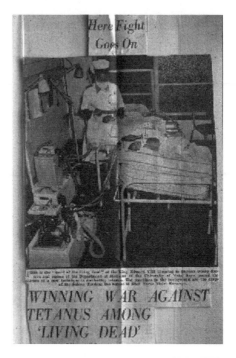

Figure 9.8 A Durban newspaper carries the story of the new treatment for tetanus in babies. (Photograph taken by Keith Sykes.)

Meanwhile, Lewis Harrington Wright was trying to persuade anaesthetists to take an interest in the drug. As we shall see in the next chapter, they took some persuading.

References

1. Blackburn J. *Charles Waterton (1782–1865). Traveller and Conservationist.* London: Vintage, 1997: 66–7.
2. Travers B. A further inquiry concerning constitutional irritation and the pathology of the nervous system. London: Longman, 1835. In Bryn Thomas K. *Curare: its history and usage.* Philadelphia: JB Lippincott, 1963.
3. Sayre LA, Burrall FA. Two cases of traumatic tetanus. *New York Journal of Medicine* 1858;**4**:250–253.
4. Wells TS. Three cases of tetanus in which 'woorara' was used. *Proceedings of the Royal Medical and Chirurgical Society (London)* 1859;**3**:142–157.
5. West R. Curare in man. *Proceedings of the Royal Society of Medicine* 1932;**25**:1107–16.

6. King H. Curare alkaloids. Part 1. Tubocurarine. *Journal of the Chemical Society* 1935;**1**:1381–9.

7. Gray TC, Halton J. A milestone in anaesthesia? (*d*-tubocurarine chloride). *Proceedings of the Royal Society of Medicine* 1946;**39**:400–8.

8. Florey HW, Harding HD, Fildes P. The treatment of tetanus. *Lancet* 1934;**ii**:1036–41.

9. Gill R. *White Water: and Black Magic*. New York: Henry Holt, 1940.

10. Gill Mrs RC. Mrs. Robinson Crusoe in Ecuador. *National Geographic Magazine* 1934;**65**:133–72.

11. Humble RM. The Gill–Merrill expedition. Penultimate chapter in the curare story. *Anesthesiology* 1982;**57**:519–26.

12. Bennett AE. How 'Indian arrow poison' curare became a useful drug. *Anesthesiology* 1967;**28**:446–52.

13. Wintersteiner O, Dutcher JD. Curare alkaloids from *Chondodendron tomentosum*. *Science* 1943;**97**:467–70.

14. Palmer H. The use of curare with convulsion therapy. *Journal of Mental Science* 1946;**92**:411–13.

15. Drinker P, Shaw LA. An apparatus for the prolonged administration of artificial respiration. 1. A design for adults and children. *Journal of Clinical Investigation* 1929;**7**:229–47.

16. Turner VC, Galloway TC. Tetanus treated as a respiratory problem. *Archives of Surgery (Chicago)* 1949;**58**:478–83.

17. Woolmer R, Cates JE. Succinylcholine in the treatment of tetanus. *Lancet* 1952;**ii**:808–9.

18. Lassen HCA, Bjørnboe M, Ibsen B, Neukirch F. Treatment of tetanus with curarisation, general anaesthesia, and intra-tracheal positive pressure ventilation. *Lancet* 1954;**ii**:1040–4.

19. Honey GE, Dwyer BE, Smith AC, Spalding JMK. Tetanus treated with tubocurarine and intermittent positive-pressure respiration. *British Medical Journal* 1954;**ii**:442–3.

20. Smythe PM, Bull A. Treatment of tetanus neonatorum with intermittent positive pressure respiration. *British Medical Journal* 1959;**ii**:107–13.

21. Wriqht R, Sykes MK, Jackson BG, Mann NM, Adams EB. Intermittent positive pressure respiration in tetanus neonatorum. *Lancet* 1961;**ii**:678–80.

22. Adams EB, Holloway R, Thambiran AK, Desai SO. Usefulness of intermittent positive pressure respiration in the treatment of tetanus. *Lancet* 1966;**ii**:1176–81.

10 Curare transforms anaesthesia

The use of curare transformed anaesthetic practice. Anaesthesia and muscle relaxation could now be induced quickly, and side-effects were minimal. Why, then, was its introduction delayed for so long?

François Magendie and some of the early physiologists who were working before anaesthesia was discovered used curare to keep animals still during experiments, and it was not until the end of the 19th century that they began to anaesthetize the animal before giving the muscle relaxant. The physiologists did, however, recognize that it was necessary to provide artificial ventilation when the animal was paralysed by curare. The early devices used to support ventilation, although ingenious, were relatively inefficient. As already mentioned in Chapter 3, it was Janeway and Green in America who first clearly demonstrated the effectiveness of intermittent positive-pressure ventilation. Then, in 1926, the English physiologist EH Starling described a piston pump that could be connected to a tracheostomy tube that provided an airtight connection with the animal's lungs. Although the pump proved to be very reliable, over a decade was to elapse before the Swedish surgeon Clarence Crafoord started to use a mechanical device to ventilate the lungs during thoracic surgery.[1]

Early trials in anaesthetized patients

The first attempt to produce muscle relaxation by giving curare to patients undergoing anaesthesia was made by Arthur Läwen, a Leipzig surgeon. In 1912, he described how he used small doses to relax the muscles during closure of the abdomen, but commented that he could not obtain enough of the crude preparation to enable him to determine an appropriate dose.[2] The second person to use curare in anaesthesia was

FP De Caux, an adventurous London anaesthetist, who administered a crude preparation in 1928 but failed to publish his observations.[3] As is so often the case in medicine, these early observations were only unearthed in recent years, and were not known to those working with curare in the 1940s.

Most of the credit for the introduction of curare into anaesthesia should go to Lewis Wright, a physician working for the pharmaceutical company ER Squibb in the USA (Figure 10.1). He had been trained as an anaesthetist in Emery E Rovenstine's department in New York. He believed that curare had a potential use in anaesthesia, and worked hard to interest other anaesthetists in its use.[4] One of those approached by Wright was Stuart Cullen, an anaesthetist in Iowa City and later Chairman of the Department of Anesthesia and Dean of the University of California Medical School in San Francisco (Figure 10.2). Responding to Wright's invitation in 1940, Cullen tested an early preparation of curare in dogs and noted salivation, extreme respiratory depression and asphyxial movements with doses adequate for abdominal relaxation. Not surprisingly, he decided not to use the drug in patients.[5]

The effects of the crude drug were further investigated by EM Papper at New York University and Bellevue Hospital in New York City. At that

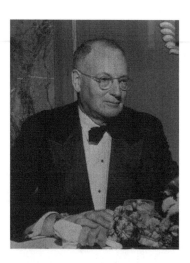

Figure 10.1 Lewis H Wright, who was instrumental in persuading Harold Griffith to use curare in the anaesthetized patient. (Reproduced with kind permission from the Wood Library–Museum of Anesthesiology, Park Ridge, Illinois.)

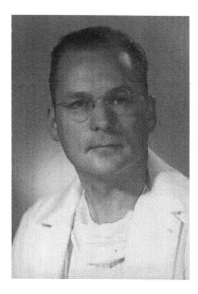

Figure 10.2 Stuart C Cullen, who initially decided not to use curare in humans because of side-effects noted in animal experiments. (Reproduced with kind permission from the Wood Library–Museum of Anesthesiology, Park Ridge, Illinois.)

time, Papper was a junior member of the Department of Anaesthesia, although he later became a distinguished Chairman of the Anaesthesia Department at the Columbia–Presbyterian Hospital in New York City (Figure 10.3). In Bellevue, the common experimental animals were monkeys and cats. Monkeys were deemed to be too expensive, so the preparation was given to two cats, both of which died from what appeared to be an acute attack of asthma.[6] Despite such unpromising results, the Chairman of the Department, Emery Rovenstine, suggested that Papper should try the drug in humans. The drug was given to two patients anaesthetized with ether, since this was the agent most commonly used at that time. Both patients developed such prolonged respiratory paralysis that their ventilation had to be supported by manually compressing the anaesthetic reservoir bag overnight. Since respiratory arrest was not then regarded with the same equanimity as it is today, the trial was abandoned. With such dramatic failures in animals and patients, it seemed unlikely that curare would prove useful in clinical

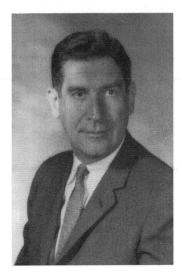

Figure 10.3 Emanuel Papper (1915–2002), who abandoned the use of curare after administering it to two patients. (Reproduced with kind permission from the Wood Library–Museum of Anesthesiology, Park Ridge, Illinois.)

practice. But a Canadian anaesthetist, Harold Randall Griffith, thought otherwise (Figure 10.4).

Harold Griffith

Griffith was born in Montreal in 1894, the son of a practitioner of homeopathic medicine.[7] When he was 16 years old, he enrolled on a combined course in arts and medicine, studying such diverse subjects as English literature, geology and genetics, as well as basic medical subjects. In 1914, he and a number of student colleagues enrolled in the Sixth Field Ambulance, which became part of the Canadian Expeditionary Force. He served as a stretcher-bearer in France, was involved in the terrible battles of the Somme and the capture of Vimy Ridge, and was awarded the Military Medal for bravery. In 1917, he transferred to the Royal Navy and served in the Mediterranean as a temporary probationer–surgeon. Griffith returned to Montreal in 1918 and survived the influenza epidemic that killed more people worldwide than had been killed in the war. He graduated in 1922, spent a year studying homeopathic medicine at the Hahnemann College in

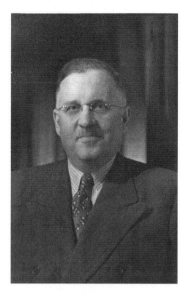

Figure 10.4 Harold Randall Griffith (1894–1985), who introduced curare into anaesthetic practice in 1942. (Reproduced with kind permission from the Wood Library–Museum of Anesthesiology, Park Ridge, Illinois.)

Philadelphia, and then entered general practice with his father. Griffith succeeded his father as superintendent of the Homeopathic Hospital in 1936, but by that time he had become a full-time anaesthetist.

Griffith was one of the anaesthetists who was approached by Wright. He was aware that Bennett had been using curare to reduce the severity of the spasms produced by convulsive therapy in psychiatric patients. More importantly, he was confident of his ability to cope with the main problem likely to arise from its use, namely respiratory paralysis. Griffith later wrote:

> *'I met Dr Wright again in 1941, and asked him how he was getting along with his idea. He said he still thought that curare might be of value to the anaesthetist but he hadn't been able to get anyone to try it in the Operating Room. I argued to myself that if it did not kill Dr Bennett's patients it could hardly do any harm to ours, because the major danger would be respiratory paralysis and even at that time anaesthetists were accustomed to maintaining controlled respiration over long periods, so I asked Dr Wright to send me some Intocostrin'.*[8]

It was in July 1942 that Griffith and his colleague Enid Johnson reported their successful use of Intocostrin in 25 patients who were lightly anaesthetized with the gas cyclopropane. Their paper transformed the practice of anaesthesia, for it demonstrated that muscular relaxation could now be achieved quickly and without the need for deep anaesthesia.[9] Cullen soon realized that he had missed a golden opportunity, and within a year he reported that he had used Intocostrin in 131 anaesthetized patients.[10] Then, in 1944, Ralph Waters of Madison, Wisconsin reported that it was not necessary to give a potent general anaesthetic and that curare worked perfectly well when combined with light nitrous oxide anaesthesia.[11] This technique eliminated the side-effects associated with potent inhalation agents and at the same time promoted a rapid recovery.

Waters' observation proved to be the key to the future popularity of the drug, but it soon became apparent that nitrous oxide was not sufficiently potent to maintain unconsciousness and analgesia in all patients. In 1947, William Neff in San Francisco described how some patients anaesthetized with nitrous oxide and curare grimaced or displayed an increase in pulse rate and blood pressure when the abdominal viscera were handled.[12] He interpreted this as being a response to pain and found that it was prevented by the intravenous injection of morphine or pethidine (meperidine; Demerol). Intravenous analgesia became very popular, and is still used today, although with shorter-acting and more effective analgesic drugs.

Curare comes to Britain

In 1943, John Halton, an innovative Liverpool anaesthetist who was at the time serving in the Royal Air Force, persuaded an American friend from a bomber squadron stationed nearby to bring some Intocostrin from the USA. Halton and Cecil Gray, later Professor in Liverpool, used the drug on patients, and were so impressed with the results that they decided to conduct a full-scale clinical trial (Figure 10.5). Supplies of Intocostrin were limited, however, so they began to use the purified preparation d-tubocurarine in their clinical practice. By 1946, they were able to report on its successful use in 1000 anaesthetics.[13]

Another person who obtained some Intocostrin was Helen Barnes, an anaesthetist in the Emergency Medical Service in London.[14] In a remarkable letter published in *The Lancet* of 1943, she reported that after reading about the use of Intocostrin to reduce the severity of the pentylenetetrazole (Metrazol) convulsions used in psychiatry, she thought the drug might relax the laryngeal muscles and so facilitate

(a) 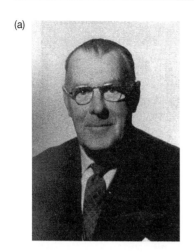 (b)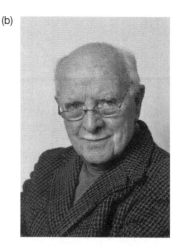

Figure 10.5 (a) John Halton (1903–1968), who obtained the first supplies of Intocostrin to be used in Liverpool. (Reproduced from Gray TC. Luck was a lady. In: Atkinson RS, Boulton TB, eds. *The History of Anaesthesia*. London: Royal Society of Medicine, 1989; 2.5 18.) (b) T Cecil Gray (1913–), who conducted the first major trials of the use of curare in Liverpool with John Halton. (Reproduced by kind permission of the University of Liverpool, Department of Anaesthesia.)

intubation of the trachea.[14] To test its efficacy, she had asked two of her colleagues to give her an intravenous injection of 4 ml of Intocostrin. After the experiment, she wrote:

> *'My sensations were dramatic. I feel that I experienced the sufferings of a patient with myasthenia gravis. At once my vision became blurred and I almost "blacked out"; then came diplopia which persisted for two hours, except when a great effort to concentrate was made. Ptosis was also very oppressive, and was accompanied by extreme prostration, fatigue, a sense of impending death, and a transient sensation of constriction in the throat'.[14]*

She noted that her colleagues had been able to pass a laryngoscope and observe her vocal cords with great ease, even though she was fully conscious at the time. As a result of these observations, she recommended the use of Intocostrin for viewing the larynx, and reported that tubes had been inserted into the trachea in five patients with the aid of the drug. It is remarkable that Helen Barnes should have volunteered for such an experiment so soon after the introduction of Intocostrin into anaesthetic practice.

The voluntary muscles vary in their sensitivity to curare, the eye muscles being the most sensitive and the diaphragm the least, so anaesthetists initially used small doses of *d*-tubocurarine that produced moderate abdominal muscle relaxation, but allowed some spontaneous movement of the diaphragm to continue. To ensure that adequate ventilation was maintained, they assisted respiration by compressing the reservoir bag synchronously with the patient's spontaneous breathing. It soon became apparent that the muscle relaxant produced very few side-effects, so doses were increased. This resulted in complete respiratory paralysis. It then became necessary for anaesthetists to assume full control of ventilation, which they attempted to do at a rate and depth that was approximately the same as the patient's normal spontaneous respiration. At this time, there were no methods of measuring whether ventilation was adequate or not, so the anaesthetist tended to give rather larger and more frequent breaths than normal, and in 1952 Gray and Rees claimed that hyperventilation enabled smaller quantities of drugs to be used.[15] It was also common practice to give 30% oxygen in the gas mixture to ensure that the patient was well oxygenated. With these precautions, it was rare for the patient to suffer respiratory problems during surgery.

But problems did arise in the postoperative period if the patient had been given too much curare and the anaesthetist had failed to ensure that its action had been completely reversed by the injection of the antagonist neostigmine. It was soon discovered that there were a number of factors that could affect the patient's sensitivity to curare and that failure to reduce the dose in these circumstances might lead to a prolonged period of respiratory inadequacy after operation.[16] A failure to appreciate the significance of these observations may have accounted for some of the excessive mortality associated with its early use in American teaching hospitals (discussed below).

The problem of consciousness in the paralysed patient

In the early trials, some anaesthetists gained the impression that curare also produced unconsciousness. For example, in 1945, RJ Whitacre and AJ Fisher in the USA reported that they had given double the normal dose of Intocostrin to patients and that surgery had been performed without any other anaesthetic agent.[17] Alarmingly, two out of the five patients reported excruciating pain. Scott Smith in Salt Lake City also began to use curare without any other anaesthetic agent in babies who were severely ill, his reason for doing so being the belief that such patients would not survive if given a general anaesthetic drug. He noted that the paralysed infants did not move when subjected to surgery and wrongly concluded that curare also had an anaesthetic effect. These conclusions were strongly contested by Louis S Goodman, the Professor of Pharmacology at the University of Utah and coauthor of the most authoritative textbook on pharmacology.

To resolve this problem, 'the intrepid Scott Smith' (as he became known subsequently) offered himself as an experimental subject. He received approximately three times the normal dose of curare while being artificially ventilated by a bag and facemask. He remained conscious throughout the experiment. His graphic description of the experience, published in 1947, convinced most anaesthetists that curare did not produce unconsciousness.[18] It also confirmed the 1946 report by the pharmacologist Frederick Prescott and the Westminster Hospital anaesthetists Geoffrey Organe and Stanley Rowbotham that described how Prescott had submitted himself to a similar experiment using Intocostrin.[19] Prescott subsequently stated that the experience was so harrowing that he never wanted to go through it again.

Although anaesthetists now know that curare is not an anaesthetic, there have been a number of occasions when a patient has been paralysed by curare or another muscle relaxant drug but has not received enough anaesthesia to produce unconsciousness. Other patients may have been conscious but have not suffered pain because they were receiving an analgesic drug such as nitrous oxide. On rare occasions, a patient may, by mistake, have received only oxygen and suffered the pain of operation without being able to move. One such patient, undergoing major surgery at a time when curare had only recently been introduced, reported to her anaesthetist postoperatively:

'I remember going to sleep after your injection into my arm, but some time later was wakened by the most excruciating pain in my tummy. It felt as if my whole insides were being pulled out; I wanted to cry but I couldn't move any part of me. I heard the doctors talking about the gallbladder, then I went to sleep again'.[20]

The patient probably experienced pain because of an interruption in the supply of nitrous oxide. Fortunately, patients are most unlikely to undergo a similar experience today, because the concentration of the inspired gases is continuously monitored and there are alarms that warn the anaesthetist of any deviation from normal settings, but in earlier days there were no such instruments and, if the anaesthetist was busy pumping blood into the patient, it was easy to miss the emptying of a gas cylinder.

The problem of assessing the depth of anaesthesia remains with us today, for it may be necessary to employ the lightest levels of anaesthesia to minimize the effects on the circulation and to ensure that patients recover quickly. There are now instruments that measure the electrical activity of the brain as an index of depth of anaesthesia, but these are not completely reliable. Whereas there are few difficulties in establishing the depth of a general anaesthetic such as ether, it is much more difficult to determine whether a patient is unconscious when extremely light anaesthesia is being used.[21] Despite these difficulties, the incidence of awareness is very low (about 0.2%). The complication is most likely to occur when the anaesthetist is forced to give a high concentration of oxygen to sustain life in an emergency situation and in so doing has to reduce the concentration of nitrous oxide.

'Balanced anaesthesia'

Although Macintosh in Oxford[22] and Forrester in Glasgow[23] were the first to report on the use of curare in anaesthesia in the UK, it was Cecil Gray and John Halton of Liverpool who popularized the use of the drug by reintroducing the term 'balanced anaesthesia'.[24] This concept was originally proposed in 1911 by George Washington Crile of Cleveland, and later modified by John Lundy at the Mayo Clinic.[25] With the modern relaxant technique, the three components of general anaesthesia – unconsciousness, analgesia and muscle relaxation – are produced by separate agents. Unconsciousness is induced by the intravenous injection of a drug such as thiopental (Pentothal) and maintained with inhalation of nitrous oxide and oxygen. Nitrous oxide also provides analgesia, but this often needs to be augmented by adding a small concentration of one of the newer volatile agents such as isoflurane or by injecting a narcotic drug. The resulting light level of anaesthesia is suitable for most operations on the body surface, and the patient will continue to breathe spontaneously, provided that narcotic overdose is avoided. But if the surgeon needs muscular relaxation, the anaesthetist will inject one of the newer synthetic muscle relaxant drugs and either assist or control the ventilation.

This technique enables the anaesthetist to induce anaesthesia rapidly, produces few side- or after-effects, and results in rapid recovery from anaesthesia. Its widespread use has revolutionized anaesthesia and has enabled surgeons to undertake more complicated surgery. Jackson Rees

(Figure 10.6), in Liverpool, developed a similar technique for use in newborn babies and children, and this has proved so successful that it has been taken up worldwide.[26] The introduction of this technique has enabled neonatal and paediatric surgery to develop in a way that would not have been possible with earlier techniques of anaesthesia.

But is curare safe?

By the 1950s, curare was being used routinely in many parts of the world, so the anaesthetic community was shattered when, in 1954, Henry Beecher and Donald Todd at the Massachusetts General Hospital in Boston published a study that revealed that the surgical mortality in patients given curare was five to six times higher than in patients not given a muscle relaxant drug. The study analysed the deaths associated with anaesthesia and surgery in ten North American University Hospitals over a five-year period up to the end of 1952.[27] The planning and organization of this study was a major achievement, for it involved the collection and analysis of mortality data on some 599 548 anaesthetics. This sample was believed to represent about 2.5% of all the anaesthetics given in all the voluntary, non-profit hospitals in the USA.

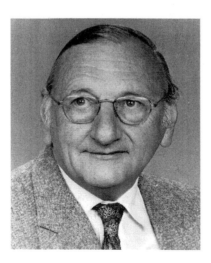

Figure 10.6 G Jackson Rees (1918–2001), the Liverpool paediatric anaesthetist who developed the use of curare in neonates and children. (Reproduced by kind permission of the University of Liverpool, Department of Anaesthesia.)

The paper produced an uproar among the anaesthetic community in the USA, and incredulity elsewhere, for many anaesthetists had been using curare without apparent harm.[28] Another feature of the report that amazed anaesthetists was that Beecher, whose main interest was pharmacological research, had suggested that the increased death rate might have been due to some inherent toxicity of the drug. It had been known since 1946 that curare could release histamine and that this could cause a decrease in blood pressure, but this phenomenon was usually accompanied by other signs of an allergic reaction and was not a common occurrence. There were no other obvious signs of drug toxicity, so there seemed to be little evidence to support Beecher's suggestion. The debate about the significance of the study went on for several years, but anaesthetists continued to use curare and the newly introduced short-acting muscle relaxant suxamethonium (succinylcholine; Anectine, Scoline).

There can be no doubt about the validity of the results. It seems to those of us who lived through this period that the most likely cause of death was a failure to secure the airway at the beginning of the anaesthetic, and a failure to ensure that the patient was breathing adequately at the end of the operation. Most American anaesthetists had been taught to intubate under deep ether anaesthesia, and although the view of the larynx under ether anaesthesia was not as good as with curare, the use of ether did ensure that spontaneous ventilation was maintained throughout the procedure. Problems with regurgitation of stomach contents during induction of anaesthesia with thiopental and curare had been noted in the preliminary reports of the Association of Anaesthetists' study of mortality.[29,30] so it seems likely that the increased mortality was due to a lack of experience with the drug and a failure to apply the basic rules concerning the maintenance of the airway and provision of adequate ventilation.

The problem of postoperative respiratory inadequacy was also greater with curare. One of the advantages of ether was that it only depressed respiration in the deepest planes of anaesthesia. Postoperative respiratory depression was therefore rarely seen, unless an opiate drug had been given for pain relief. Curare, on the other hand, produced progressive paralysis of the respiratory muscles, so the diaphragm could produce some breathing activity even when the other respiratory muscles were still paralysed. Anaesthetists and recovery room staff were not aware of the dangers of partial respiratory paralysis, and the use of neostigmine to reverse the paralysis at the end of the operation was not common practice in the USA at that time.

The problem of residual paralysis and chest complications was later highlighted in a study comparing ether anaesthesia with a technique employing a continuous infusion of the short-acting relaxant, suxamethonium. This showed a higher incidence of pulmonary complications in the group receiving the muscle relaxant.[31]

To summarize:

By 1946, 100 years after Morton gave the first ether anaesthetic for a surgical operation, anaesthetists at last had the tools that enabled them to provide an ideal anaesthetic. Anaesthesia could be induced rapidly and pleasantly, ideal operating conditions could be produced with few undesirable side-effects, and recovery was rapid, with significantly fewer postoperative complications. But the ability to provide a smooth anaesthetic was not enough to establish anaesthesia as a speciality in its own right. Anaesthesia had to develop a scientific background. It did so initially by astute observation and experimentation in the clinical environment. It was not until the 1950s that laboratory investigations began to provide a true scientific basis for the speciality.

References

1. Frenckner P, Andersson E, Crafoord P. A new and practical method of producing rhythmic ventilation during positive pressure anaesthesia. *Acta Otolaryngologica* 1940;**28**:95–102.
2. Läwen A. Ueber die verbindung der localanästhesie mit der narcose, über hohe extraduralanästhesie und epidurale injectionen anästhesierender lösungen bei tabischen magenkrisen. *Beiträge zur klinischen Chirurgie* 1912;**80**:168–189.
3. Wilkinson DJ. Dr. F.P. de Caux – the first user of curare for anaesthesia in England. *Anaesthesia* 1991;**46**:49–51.
4. Betcher AM. The civilising of curare: a history of its development and introduction into anesthesiology. *Anesthesia and Analgesia* 1977;**56**:305–19.
5. Bennett AE. How 'Indian arrow poison' curare became a useful drug. *Anesthesiology* 1967;**28**:446–52.
6. Papper EM. The friend of the young anaesthetist. *Canadian Journal of Anaesthesia* 1992;**39**:(Suppl): 9–10.
7. Bodman R, Gillies D. *Harold Griffith. The Evolution of Modern Anaesthesia.* Toronto and Oxford: Dundurn Press, 1992.
8. Maltby JR, Shephard DAE, eds. Harold Griffith: His Life and Legacy. *Canadian Journal of Anaesthesia* 1992;**39**(Suppl): 4.
9. Griffith HR, Johnson GE. The use of curare in general anesthesia. *Anesthesiology* 1942;**3**:418–20.
10. Cullen SC. The use of curare for the improvement of abdominal muscle relaxation during inhalation anesthesia. Report on one hundred and thirty one cases. *Surgery* 1943;**14**:261–6.
11. Waters RM. Nitrous oxide–oxygen and curare. *Anesthesiology* 1944;**5**:618–19.

12. Neff W, Mayer EC, de la Luz Perales M. Nitrous oxide and oxygen anesthesia with curare relaxation. *California Medicine* 1947;**66**:67–9.

13. Gray TC, Halton J. A milestone in anaesthesia? (*d*-tubocurarine chloride). *Proceedings of the Royal Society of Medicine* 1946;**39**:400–8.

14. Barnes H. Use of curare for direct oral intubation. *Lancet* 1943;**i**:478.

15. Gray TC, Rees GJ. The role of apnoea for major surgery. *British Medical Journal* 1952;**ii**:891–2.

16. Feldman S. *Poison Arrows*. London: Metro Publishing, 2005: 132.

17. Whitacre RJ, Fisher AJ. Clinical observations on the use of curare in anesthesia. *Anesthesiology* 1945;**6**:124–30.

18. Smith SM, Brown HO, Toman JEP, Goodman LS. The lack of cerebral effects of *d*-tubocurarine. *Anesthesiology* 1947;**8**:1–14.

19. Prescott F, Organe G, Rowbotham S. Tubocurarine as an adjunct to anaesthesia. Report on 180 cases. *Lancet* 1946;**ii**:80–4.

20. Winterbottom EH. Insufficent anaesthesia. *British Medical Journal* 1950;**i**:247–8.

21. Sandin RH, Enlund G, Samuelsson P, Lennmarken C. Awareness during anaesthesia: a prospective case study. *Lancet* 2000;**355**:707–11.

22. Macintosh RR. Curare in anaesthesia. *Lancet* 1945;**ii**:124.

23. Forrester AC. Curare in anaesthesia: report of 100 cases. *Glasgow Medical Journal* 1946;**27**:211–19.

24. Gray TC, Halton J. Technique for the use of d-tubocurarine chloride with balanced anaesthesia. *British Medical Journal* 1946;**ii**:293–5.

25. Lundy JS. Balanced anesthesia. *Survey of Anesthesiology* 1981;**25**:272–8.

26. Rees GJ. Anaesthesia in the newborn. *British Medical Journal* 1950;**ii**:1419–22.

27. Beecher HK, Todd DP. A study of the deaths associated with anesthesia and surgery. *Annals of Surgery* 1954;**140**:2–34.

28. Abajian J, Arrowood JG, Bartlett RH et al. A critique of 'A study of the deaths associated with anesthesia and surgery'. *Annals of Surgery* 1955;**142**:138–41. Beecher HK, Donald DP. Comment on the critique 142–4.

29. Morton HJV, Wylie WD. Anaesthetic deaths due to regurgitation. *Anaesthesia* 1951;**6**:190–201 and 205.

30. Committee on Deaths Associated with Anaesthesia. Report on 400 cases. *Anaesthesia* 1952;**7**:200–5.

31. Bunker J, Bendixen HH, Sykes MK, Todd DP, Surtees AD. A comparison of ether anesthesia with thiopental–nitrous oxide–succinylcholine for upper abdominal surgery. *Anesthesiology* 1959;**20**:745–52.

Further reading

Gray TC, Wilson F. The development and use of muscle relaxants in the United Kingdom. *Anesthesiology* 1959;**10**:519–29.

McIntyre AR. Curare. *Its History, Nature and Clinical Use*. Chicago: University of Chicago Press, 1947.

Sykes MK. The Griffith legacy. *Canadian Journal of Anaesthesia* 1993;**40**:365–74.

Thomas KB. *Curare. Its History and Usage*. Philadelphia: JB Lippincott, 1963.

Part 3

New horizons: the scientific background to anaesthesia and the emergence of intensive care

In countries that had suffered in the Second World War, there was an immense desire to create a better world. The wartime experience had broadened many people's horizons, and doctors at last had drugs, such as the sulphonamides and penicillin, that actually cured disease. These drugs, together with the later technical advances such as the introduction of plastic syringes and intravenous equipment, developments in the electronic field, and new diagnostic techniques, provided opportunities to develop new forms of treatment. In Britain, the introduction of a National Health Service, free to all, in 1948, provided an unrivalled opportunity to create a new style of medicine. Anaesthetists were at last recognized as Consultants with the same status as Consultants in medicine, surgery and the other specialities, and they now had the technical capability to anaesthetize patients quickly and safely for the new operations that surgeons were developing. The scientific background to anaesthesia was being established by research, and drug firms were beginning to introduce new additions to the anaesthetist's armamentarium. The next half-century saw a revolution in anaesthetic practice, both in the operating room and elsewhere in the hospital. We now document this explosion of activity.

11 'Physiological trespass': the reduction of surgical bleeding and the control of other body systems

Surgeons have always recognized that bleeding is an inevitable consequence of surgery, but they were astonished when, in 1948, the Edinburgh anaesthetists HWC Griffith and John Gillies reported that they had deliberately reduced blood pressure to unrecordable levels to allow James Learmonth, Professor of Surgery, to operate with a bloodless field. The operation, which had been designed to reduce chronic hypertension, failed to do so, but the 'physiological trespass' in which the anaesthetists engaged was a brilliant success. It opened doors for new advances in surgical technique and it radically altered the understanding of how the circulation is controlled.

Edinburgh 1948

The patients upon whom Learmonth wished to operate had persistently high blood pressures, and there were, at that time, no drugs that could be used to treat the hypertension. Surgery offered the possibility of relief by removing the sympathetic nerves that caused constriction of the blood vessels, but the operation of thoracolumbar sympathectomy entailed a major incision to allow the surgeon access to the nerves within the chest, and this had resulted in heavy blood loss. An added complication was that the operation had to be performed on each side of the chest, usually with a two-week interval between procedures. Griffith and Gillies offered to help.

Anaesthetists were aware that there was often a moderate fall in blood pressure during ordinary spinal anaesthesia and that this decreased blood loss during surgery. The decrease in blood pressure during spinal anaesthesia had been considered a serious and unwanted complication in the past, but Griffith and Gillies intended to make it an asset. The radical solution they adopted was to render the patient unconscious with a large dose of thiopental and then to administer a local anaesthetic drug to achieve *total* spinal anaesthesia. The local anaesthetic solution not only blocked all the nerves carrying pain impulses from the chest and the abdomen, but also blocked the transmission of nerve impulses in the sympathetic nerves as they left the spinal cord. The sympathetic nerve block resulted in a dilatation of the smaller arteries and a dramatic decrease in blood pressure. Indeed, the blood pressure fell to such low levels that it could not be recorded with the usual methods; the only signs of life were the weak heart beats that could be felt in the chest, and regular spontaneous breathing that showed that the vital centres in the brain were still receiving an adequate blood supply. Not surprisingly, there was scarcely any bleeding from the surgical field, thus allowing the surgeon to complete the operation within the hour. Since blood loss was minimal, the patient's recovery was more rapid than would otherwise have been the case. King George VI subsequently underwent similar surgery in 1949, and on this occasion Learmonth was joined by the London surgeon, Professor James Paterson Ross. Both surgeons were knighted for their efforts.

The concept of *induced* or *controlled hypotension* required a remarkable readjustment in thinking for anaesthetists, since their whole training had been geared to maintaining blood pressure at the normal level. The idea of deliberately reducing the blood pressure to such an extent that it could no longer be recorded with the standard blood pressure cuff seemed foolhardy in the extreme; but to use the technique in patients with high blood pressure and an increased risk of coronary heart disease or stroke seemed the height of folly. In 1948, Griffith and Gillies reported that they had given 88 such anaesthetics, and that the one death in the series was due to a failure to recognize that the patient had a decreased arterial oxygen saturation resulting from a residual effusion of fluid into the chest after the first operation.[1] Were they lucky or was there a reason for the low mortality? To answer this question it is necessary to go back to 1946.

Bleeding and a brain tumour

In that year, the American neurosurgeon WJ Gardner was faced with the problem of removing a very large vascular tumour of the brain. He was worried that the patient might die from excessive bleeding, and eventually decided that the safest course of action would be to bleed the patient into a reservoir until the blood pressure had fallen to a low level, remove the tumour, and then reinfuse the blood at the end of the operation. In fact, Gardner only reduced the systolic blood pressure from 160 to 100 mmHg, but this reduced the bleeding so that he was able to remove the tumour successfully.[2]

Gardner did, however, recognize that the bleeding had created a state of surgical or haemorrhagic shock. In this type of shock, the loss of blood decreases the venous pressure so that less blood returns to the heart. This leads to a decrease in cardiac output and a fall in arterial pressure, in response to which the arterioles and veins constrict in an attempt to return the blood pressure to normal levels. Gardner recognized that it was probably the compensatory vasoconstriction that had been the most important factor in decreasing the bleeding in his patient. But he also recognized that the severe decrease in cardiac output and vasoconstriction might deprive vital organs of their blood supply and that this might lead to the onset of irreversible shock, a dreaded complication at that time when little was known about the physiology of shock.[3] Subsequently, Donald E Hale at the Cleveland Clinic used a similar technique in some 50 patients who were undergoing neurosurgical operations and fenestration operations for deafness, but the practice soon ceased because of concern about the blood flow to vital organs.[4]

The sympathetic nerve block accompanying total spinal anaesthesia leads to a profound reduction in blood pressure lasting for 30–40 minutes, the pressure then returning gradually to normal levels. Griffith and Gilles observed that bleeding was still minimal when the pressure had risen to 60–80 mmHg, and, since this level of pressure could be measured with the standard blood pressure cuff, thus providing some reassurance for the anaesthetist, they subsequently modified their technique so as to maintain this level of pressure throughout the operation. Over the next two or three years, Philip Bromage, one of the few English anaesthetists with an extensive experience of epidural anaesthesia (which also blocks the sympathetic nerves), used this technique to produce a blood pressure of 50–60 mmHg for a wide range of surgical procedures.[5] By 1951, however, when he published his results, specific blood pressure-lowering drugs were being introduced: since these drugs could be injected intravenously, acted rapidly and enabled a more exact control of blood pressure to be achieved, they soon replaced spinal and epidural techniques.

Blood pressure-lowering drugs

In the late 1940s, the pharmacologists WDM Paton and Eleanor J Zaimis, who were investigating the muscle-relaxant properties of new drugs, reported that two of them, hexamethonium and pentamethonium, also blocked the transmission of nerve impulses in the sympathetic ganglia and so caused dilatation of the arterioles. These drugs thus produced the same effects that Learmonth had been seeking. A number of anaesthetists then started to use these and other drugs to produce hypotension during anaesthesia.[6–10]

Within a few years better control was provided by the introduction of the short-acting drug trimetaphan (Arfonad), which not only blocked the transmission of impulses through the ganglia, but also dilated the arterioles by a direct action on the smooth muscle in their walls. Finally, anaesthetists started to use sodium nitroprusside and nitroglycerine (glyceryl trinitrate), which acted only on the muscle in the arterioles, nitroglycerine having been used to vasodilate the coronary arteries in patients with angina of effort since 1879. Since these drugs were given by intravenous infusion, the infusion rate could be adjusted on a minute-to-minute basis to provide the desired level of blood pressure reduction.[11]

Benefits and risk

Griffith and Gillies were surprised that the total spinal technique apparently caused little harm, and suggested that the safety of the technique was due to the fact that the dilatation of the blood vessels that produced the fall in blood pressure also decreased the resistance to blood flow. Thus, blood flow to the cells might be maintained despite the decrease in driving pressure. Support for their hypothesis was provided by Nicholas Greene, an anesthesiologist from the Massachusetts General Hospital in Boston, who visited Edinburgh and, on his return, initiated a series of studies on controlled hypotension. In 1954, he and his colleagues confirmed that the essential difference between a reduction in blood pressure resulting from haemorrhage and a similar reduction due to sympathetic blockade lay in the state of the arterioles. In haemorrhagic shock, cardiac output is greatly reduced and the arterioles are severely constricted in an effort to restore blood pressure to normal levels. The combination of low cardiac output and vasoconstriction causes the vital organs to be starved of blood so that the metabolic processes are disturbed. With sympathetic blockade or with the other blood pressure-lowering drugs, the arterioles are dilated and, although cardiac output may be somewhat reduced, blood flow to vital organs is relatively well maintained.[12]

Induced hypotension was initially utilized in major operations where there was significant blood loss, or in operations in which there was a risk of rupturing a blood vessel, for example in the surgery of intracranial aneurysms or in operations on the aorta. Within a few years, surgeons were requesting induced hypotension for plastic surgery on the nose and face, since they felt that they could perform a better repair when there was a bloodless field. The lack of bleeding when the surgeon made his incision was astonishing and scared many anaesthetists when they first used the technique, but they soon found that an arterial pressure of around 60 mmHg could be tolerated for several hours without apparent damage to the brain or other organs, whereas a similar period of hypotension due to blood loss would often prove fatal.

Nevertheless, Gillies admitted that the technique of induced hypotension represented 'physiological trespass', that normal safety margins were being eroded and that the technique carried an inherent risk. For example, any decrease in blood pressure will inevitably cause a decrease in blood flow if an artery is partially obstructed by disease, so patients with arterial disease may suffer a coronary thrombosis or stroke when subjected to induced hypotension. By 1953, it had become clear that the use of induced hypotension had resulted in some deaths, and as a result a more cautious approach was adopted.[13,14] The technique is now reserved for operations where there is likely to be a large blood loss (such as operations on vascular tumours or aneurysms in the brain, or where a large amount of tissue has to be removed, for example in cancer). In these circumstances, the benefits outweigh the risk.

Understanding the circulation

The importance of controlled hypotension was not simply that it minimized blood loss and provided an improved surgical field. Equally important was the greater understanding of the behaviour of the circulation that resulted from the experience gained with this technique. The anaesthetist could observe the effects of the various methods of dilating the blood vessels, and could then see how these effects were modified by changing the venous return to the heart by posture or an increased pressure within the lungs, or by changing blood volume. The new knowledge of the behaviour of the circulation has benefited many aspects of anaesthetic practice. For example, it is now common practice for the anaesthetist or intensive care doctor to use vasodilating drugs when the patient develops marked hypertension during surgery or after cardiac operations. Furthermore, patients with severe hypertension will often be treated with antihypertensive drugs preoperatively to decrease the risk of a heart attack during or after surgery. Anaesthetists have since conducted many studies that have thrown new light on the way in which patients with high blood pressure and coronary artery disease respond to anaesthesia and surgery, and these have resulted in alterations in drug therapy. This has had a significant impact on the risks of surgery in patients with arterial disease and hypertension.

The control of other body systems

There was another, and perhaps even more important, benefit resulting from the experience with induced hypotension, for it made anaesthetists realize that if they understood how a body system worked, they would be able to control it. They had already learnt to take control of the patient's ventilation. Even though, in the 1950s, they had no way of measuring whether the artificial ventilation they were providing was adequate or not, clinical experience had clearly demonstrated that the majority of patients were benefiting from the new technique. Now they realized that they could control blood pressure by manipulating the resistance of the smaller arterioles and other aspects of the circulation, and that this enabled surgeons to extend the range of surgery.

Then, in the early 1950s, physiologists, anaesthetists and surgeons started to learn how to control body temperature so that the brain could be protected during short periods of zero blood flow during cardiac and neurological surgery. It was found that induced hypothermia – a decrease in body temperature from 37°C to 30°C – could halve the brain's oxygen consumption and so double the time without blood flow (see Chapter 15). Only in the last decade has it become apparent that the maintenance of a normal body temperature during routine surgery is of equal importance. All patients tend to lose heat in the air-conditioned environment of the operating theatre, and shivering often occurs after operation. Active warming of patients on the operating table not only decreases the incidence of postoperative shivering and its deleterious effects on metabolism, but also reduces the incidence of postoperative wound infection.

Anaesthetists have also learnt how to control acid–base and electrolyte balance and various metabolic disturbances, and, as they have become increasingly involved in intensive care, they have learnt how to cope with single and multiple organ failure.

The anaesthetist has thus become a clinical scientist who is conversant with the acute disturbances of body function that occur not only during surgery or other types of trauma, but also in a wide range of acute medical conditions. By integrating recent developments in both physiology and pharmacology into their clinical practice, anaesthetists have transformed their role in medicine and provided a new perspective in the care of the acutely ill patient. Controlled hypotension initiated the change, but, as we shall see in the next chapter, it was the Copenhagen poliomyelitis epidemic of 1952 that provided the major impetus for change.

References

1. Griffiths HWC, Gillies J. Thoraco-lumbar splanchnicectomy and sympathectomy: anaesthetic procedure. *Anaesthesia* 1948;**3**:134–46.
2. Gardner WJ. The control of bleeding during operation by induced hypotension. *Journal of the American Medical Association* 1946;**132**:572–4.
3. Page IH. Vascular mechanisms of terminal shock. *Cleveland Clinic Quarterly* 1946;**13**:1–8.
4. Hale DE. Controlled hypotension by arterial bleeding during operation and anesthesia. *Anesthesiology* 1948;**9**:498–505.
5. Bromage PR. Vascular hypotension in 107 cases of epidural analgesia. *Anaesthesia* 1951;**6**:26–9.
6. Organe G, Paton WDM, Zaimis EJ. Preliminary trials of bistrimethylammonium decane and pentane iodide (C10 and C5) in man. *Lancet* 1949;**i**:21–3.
7. Davidson MHA. Pentamethonium iodide in anaesthesia. *Lancet* 1950;**i**:252–3.
8. Scurr CF. Reduction of haemorrhage in the operative field by the use of pentamethonium iodide; a preliminary report. *Anesthesiology* 1951;**12**:253–4.
9. Hunter AR. Hexamethonium bromide. *Lancet* 1950;**i**:251–2.
10. Enderby GEH. Controlled circulation with hypotensive drugs and posture to reduce bleeding in surgery. Preliminary results with pentamethonium iodide. *Lancet* 1950;**i**:1145–7.
11. Moraca PP, Bitte EM, Hale DE, Wasmuth CE, Pontasse L. Clinical evaluation of nitroprusside as a hypotensive agent. *Anesthesiology* 1962;**23**:193–9.
12. Greene NM, Bunker JP, Kerr WS. von Felsinger JM, Keller JW. Beecher HK. Hypotensive spinal anesthesia: respiratory, metabolic, hepatic, renal and cerebral effects. *Annals of Surgery* 1954;**140**:641–51.
13. Committee upon Deaths Associated with Anaesthesia. Deaths associated with anaesthesia. Cases in which hypotension has been used. *Anaesthesia* 1953;**8**:263–7.
14. Hampton LJ, Little DM. Complications associated with the use of 'controlled hypotension' in anesthesia. *American Medical Association Archives of Surgery* 1953;**67**:549–54.

12 The anaesthetist and the fever hospital

At the height of the 1952 poliomyelitis epidemic in Copenhagen, the Danish anaesthetist Bjørn Ibsen realized, as the attending doctors did not, that many of the paralysed patients were dying from respiratory failure. With his operating room experience, his knowledge of physiology and his technical skill, he was able to introduce a new form of treatment that subsequently became the mainstay of intensive care.

In 1951, there was a major International Congress in Copenhagen, Denmark, that was attended by most of the world's experts on poliomyelitis. In the summer of the following year, Copenhagen suffered one of the worst epidemics of the disease that has ever been recorded. Whether the experts brought a particularly virulent form of the virus to Copenhagen will never be known, but what is certain is that the Danish doctors' response to this epidemic had a major influence on the treatment of patients with respiratory paralysis due to poliomyelitis. Their efforts not only resulted in a completely new form of treatment for the disease, but also laid the foundations for the subsequent development of intensive care, the transport of severely ill patients, and the special blood analyses that are required for the care of patients with acute respiratory failure.

The Copenhagen poliomyelitis epidemic

The scale of the epidemic is difficult to imagine. There were 2899 cases in the 1.2 million citizens of Copenhagen – an attack rate of 238 per 100 000 inhabitants. This far exceeded that recorded in previous epidemics in New York in 1916, 1931 and 1944. Patients were admitted to the Blegdams Infectious Diseases Hospital at the rate of 50 per day and there was an unusually high incidence of paralysis of the muscles of the pharynx and larynx (bulbar paralysis) combined with paralysis of the respiratory and limb muscles (spinal paralysis). As a result, secretions from the mouth were inhaled into the lungs and, since the patients did not have enough muscle power to clear the airways by coughing, they soon developed collapse of areas of the lung and pneumonia. In the first three weeks of the epidemic, 31 patients with this bulbospinal paralysis had been treated in an iron lung or a cuirass ventilator, and of these 27 had died within 72 hours of admission – a mortality rate of over 80%. This reflected the previous experience of the Blegdams' doctors, for in the 10 years before this epidemic only 15 patients with this type of paralysis had survived. At that time, it was thought that death was due to an overwhelming viral infection at the base of the brain and that nothing further could be done.[1]

There were only six cuirass ventilators and one iron lung in the hospital, and these resources were obviously inadequate (Figures 12.1 and 12.2). At the end of the third week of the epidemic, Hans Christian Alexander Lassen, the Chief Physician at the Blegdams Fever Hospital (Figure 12.3), realized that this epidemic was quite unlike any that had been experienced before, and that something had to be done to cope with the huge influx of cases. But what could he do?

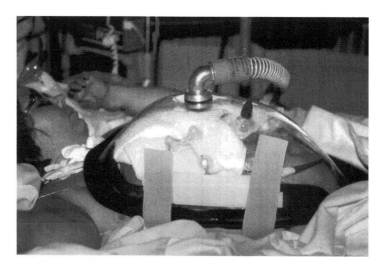

Figure 12.1 A patient with respiratory paralysis due to poliomyelitis being treated in a cuirass ventilator.

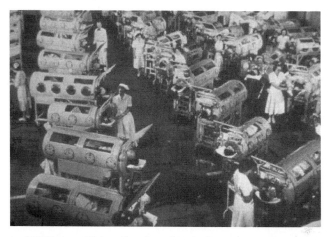

Figure 12.2 Tank ventilators ('iron lungs') in the Rancho Los Alamos Hospital, California during an outbreak of paralytic poliomyelitis in 1953. Units that specialized in the treatment of polio were the forerunners of the intensive care units of today.

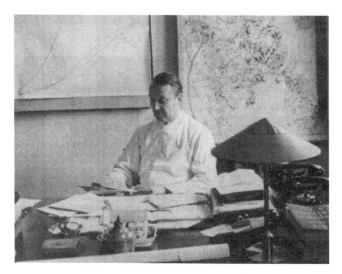

Figure 12.3 HCA Lassen, Chief Physician at Blegdams Hospital. (Reproduced with permission from Secher O. The polio epidemic in Copenhagen 1952. In: Atkinson RS, Boulton TB, eds. *The History of Anaesthesia*. London: Royal Society of Medicine, 1989: 427.)

The coincidence

It so happened that one of Lassen's staff, Mogens Bjørnboe, had travelled back from the USA by ship in 1950 and had met the wife and daughters of a Danish anaesthetist, Bjørn Ibsen, who had remained in Boston to continue his studies in the anaesthetic department at the Massachusetts General Hospital (Figure 12.4). Since anaesthesia was only just becoming established as a speciality in Denmark, Ibsen was forced to become a freelance anaesthetist when he returned to Copenhagen at the end of the year. In June 1952, while Lassen was away, a baby with tetanus had been admitted to Blegdams Hospital. With the full consent of Lassen's deputy, Fritz Neukirch, Bjørnboe asked Ibsen to advise on treatment. They decided to paralyse the baby with curare to abolish the spasms of tetanus and then to maintain breathing artificially with manually controlled ventilation, as practised in anaesthesia. The baby's condition was satisfactory when it was being ventilated by hand, but when it was returned to the usual regime where the spasms were controlled by sedation and no artificial ventilation

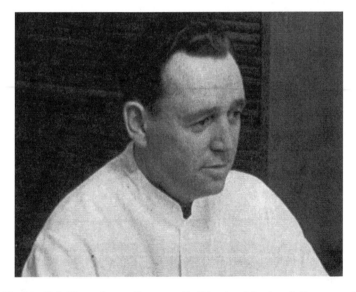

Figure 12.4 Bjørn Ibsen, the anaesthetist who introduced the use of anaesthetic techniques for treating respiratory paralysis to the fever hospital. (Reproduced with permission from Secher O. The polio epidemic in Copenhagen 1952. In: Atkinson RS, Boulton TB, eds. *The History of Anaesthesia*. London: Royal Society of Medicine, 1989: 428.)

was provided, it failed to survive. Bjørnboe had, however, been so impressed with this early trial of the new technique that he suggested to Lassen that Ibsen should be asked to help with the care of the polio patients. Lassen was in a difficult position. He was the Chief Physician in the infectious diseases hospital, and in the hierarchical medical society of the time it was not customary to take advice from any one else, much less an anaesthetist. Lassen finally realized that he had no alternative but to seek help, and invited Ibsen to a meeting on 25 August 1952.

Ibsen's background

Ibsen had spent two years at the Massachusetts General Hospital, where the Professor, Henry K Beecher, was making the first studies of blood carbon dioxide levels and acid–base balance to quantify the changes in lung function that occur during thoracic surgery.[2] Ibsen had thus become familiar with the underlying principles of gas exchange in the lung, and when he returned to Copengagen, he and a surgical colleague, HC Engell, initiated similar studies of carbon dioxide levels in expired gas in patients undergoing anaesthesia. Through this research, they learnt that inadequate ventilation of the lungs resulted in carbon dioxide retention, and that this was often associated with an increase in blood pressure and sweating. Ibsen had also read the papers of Bower and colleagues that had clearly demonstrated the importance of adequate ventilation and secretion removal in patients with bulbospinal paralysis in an American epidemic of poliomyelitis.[3,4]

When Ibsen examined patients with bulbospinal paralysis and attended the autopsies of four patients who had died from the disease, he noted that a high blood pressure and sweating had been observed in the patients shortly before death. He also noted that blood analyses taken just before death had shown a high level of 'total carbon dioxide in plasma'. This measurement was the only one available at the time, and it included all the forms in which carbon dioxide is carried in blood: as carbon dioxide gas in simple solution, carbon dioxide dissolved in water as carbonic acid, and bicarbonate ion. This measurement is affected by two factors: total carbon dioxide rises when the lungs fail to excrete the carbon dioxide produced by metabolism, but it also increases when the kidneys fail to excrete bicarbonate. In common with other physicians at the time, the physicians responsible for the polio patients' care were unfamiliar with disturbances in the physiology of the lung and assumed that the increase in total carbon dioxide was due to a retention of bicarbonate in the plasma caused by a kidney abnormality, and that this was caused by an overwhelming viral infection.[5]

165

Ibsen, who was familiar with disturbances in respiration, concluded that the children were dying from carbon dioxide retention due to respiratory failure, not to kidney failure. There were only two ways to decide which of these two alternatives was correct. One was to measure the degree of acidity or alkalinity of the blood; at that time, however, there were no commercially available pH electrodes that enabled this measurement to be made on blood samples. Ibsen therefore chose an alternative method: he decided to show that the total carbon dioxide could be returned to normal levels by increasing the ventilation artificially.

Ibsen's proposal

Ibsen proposed that a tracheostomy should be performed under local anaesthesia and a tube with an inflatable cuff should then be inserted into the trachea. This would provide an airtight seal that would enable the lungs to be ventilated with intermittent positive pressure. It would also prevent mouth secretions entering the lungs, and would enable a suction catheter to be inserted into the lower airways so that secretions could be removed and the lungs re-expanded (Figure 12.5). The tracheostomy tube was then to be connected to an anaesthetic breathing system so that the lungs could be ventilated by compression of the reservoir bag, just as was the custom during anaesthesia (Figure 12.6). Ibsen's breathing system incorporated a carbon dioxide absorber in the circuit, and the

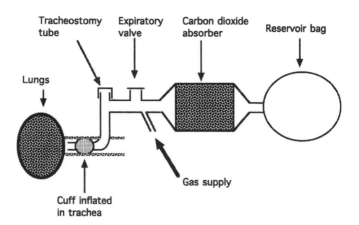

Figure 12.5 Waters breathing system with carbon dioxide absorber used to ventilate the patient through a cuffed tracheostomy tube.

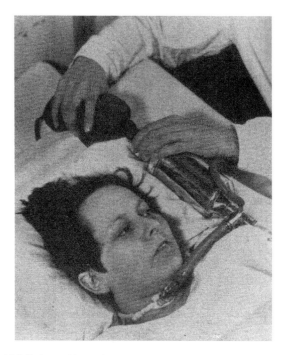

Figure 12.6 Patient with respiratory paralysis being manually ventilated with an anaesthetic breathing system. (Reproduced with permission from Secher O. The polio epidemic in Copenhagen 1952. In: Atkinson RS, Boulton TB. *The History of Anaesthesia*. London: Royal Society of Medicine, 1989: 430.)

lungs were ventilated with a 50% mixture of nitrogen and oxygen to ensure that the patient did not suffer oxygen lack if the ventilation became inadequate at any time.[6]

Lassen remained sceptical and initially rejected the plan, but two days later, on 27 August, he relented, and Ibsen was given the chance to demonstrate his therapeutic proposal in a 12-year-old girl who was close to death. She was so ill that she became unconscious during the tracheostomy operation (which was performed under local anaesthesia), and when Ibsen connected his artificial breathing system he found that he could not ventilate the lungs properly. His difficulty was probably due to spasm of the airways and collapse of part of the lungs due to the accumulation of secretions. In desperation, he gave her a small dose of intravenous thiopental to stop her struggling. She developed circulatory collapse, but he was able to ventilate the lungs. He managed to restore her circulation with a transfusion of fluids, and, when she was in a stable condition, he and his surgical research colleague HC Engell were able to show the Blegdams physicians how the carbon dioxide level could be manipulated by altering the intermittent positive pressure applied to the reservoir bag. The physicians had argued that the patients could not have been in respiratory failure because many had not been cyanosed before death. Ibsen was able to demonstrate, however, that patients breathing oxygen might not be cyanosed, even though they had a high level of carbon dioxide. Finally, the anaesthetic breathing system was disconnected and artificial ventilation was provided by the cuirass ventilator initially used for treatment. This again led to carbon dioxide retention, which could then be reversed by manual controlled ventilation. The final proof of Ibsen's diagnosis was that a blood sample taken when adequate ventilation had been restored showed a normal value for the 'total carbon dioxide in plasma'. This clearly demonstrated that the increased total carbon dioxide was due to the accumulation of carbon dioxide caused by a decrease in ventilation, and that it was not due to changes in kidney function. It was finally agreed that the cause of death in these patients was inadequate ventilation provided by the tank or cuirass ventilator when the lungs were collapsed by the accumulation of secretions.

The organization

This dramatic demonstration convinced the assembled doctors that they must switch to manual intermittent positive-pressure ventilation with the anaesthetic breathing system. The problem now became one of logistics. First, the patients requiring ventilation had to be moved to new wards so that all the necessary resources could be concentrated in one area of the hospital. Second, cuffed tracheostomy tubes, anaesthetic breathing systems and gas cylinders had to be assembled. Third, teams of internists, surgeons and anaesthetists had to be established so that they could provide skilled care throughout the 24 hours. Fortunately, the World Health Organization had set up an anaesthesia training centre in Copenhagen in 1950, so there were about 20 trainee anaesthetists who could supervise the anaesthetic care of the patients (Figure 12.7). But this was not enough: they needed people who could aspirate the secretions from the trachea and manually compress the anaesthetic reservoir bags 24 hours a day for the estimated two to three months' duration of the treatment. The Copenhagen medical students volunteered to help, and were soon organizing their own six-hour shifts. The care of these patients

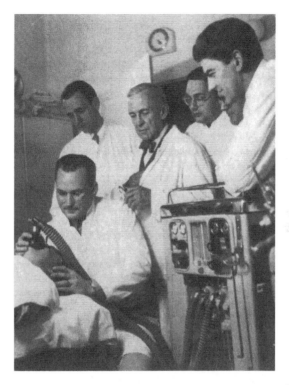

Figure 12.7 Stuart Cullen (seated) and Ralph Waters (bow-tie) demonstrating anaesthesia during the first World Health Organization course on anaesthesia in Copenhagen in 1950. Observing are Danish anaesthetists (*left to right*) Bjørn Ibsen, Henning Ruben, Erik Waino-Andersen (hidden) and Ole Secher. (Reproduced from *Acta Anaesthesiologica Scandinavica* 1990:**34**(Suppl 94), with the permission of Blackwell Publishing, Oxford.)

was a heavy responsibility, for the students not only had to aspirate secretions through the tracheostomy and maintain artificial ventilation, but also had to monitor the patient's condition and inform one of the doctors if there were problems.

At the height of the epidemic, 70 patients were being manually ventilated simultaneously. During the week from 28 August to 3 September, 335 patients were admitted to Blegdams Hospital with polio – a rate of nearly 50 per day. By November, the number of medical students was proving to be inadequate, so Lassen recruited dental students to help out. During the epidemic, approximately 1500 students put in a total of 165 000 hours ventilating patients. By the end of the epidemic, when some 800 patients had been treated, the mortality rate in patients with bulbospinal polio had been reduced from about 80% to approximately 25% – a remarkable achievement.

Within a year of the Copenhagen epidemic, a number of pioneers, including Ibsen, had created their own respiratory care units for treating poliomyelitis and other diseases such as acute polyneuritis (which also produces muscle paralysis). It was soon recognized that the Copenhagen technique enabled patients with tetanus and other convulsive conditions to be paralysed with curare and kept alive with artificial ventilation until the disease burnt itself out. By 1960, intermittent positive-pressure ventilation was being used to treat respiratory failure due to postoperative respiratory complications, trauma, head injury, drug overdose, pneumonia, acute-on-chronic bronchitis, asthma and a number of other conditions.

Today, with universal immunization, poliomyelitis has virtually disappeared in developed countries.[7] Poliomyelitis may have disappeared, but the legacy of the Copenhagen epidemic lives on in modern intensive care units, although their evolution was beset by problems.

References

1. Lassen HCA. A preliminary report on the 1952 epidemic of poliomyelitis in Copenhagen with special reference to the treatment of acute respiratory insufficiency. *Lancet* 1953;**i**:37–41.
2. Ibsen B. From anaesthesia to anaesthesiology. Personal experiences in Copenhagen during the past 25 years. *Acta Anaesthesiologica Scandinavica* 1975; **Suppl 61**.
3. Bower AG, Bennett VR, Dillon JB. Investigation on the care and treatment of poliomyelitis patients. *Annals of Western Medicine and Surgery* 1950;**4**:561–82.
4. Bower AG, Bennett VR, Dillon JB, Axelrod B. Investigation on the care and treatment of poliomyelitis patients. Part 2. Physiological studies of various treatment procedures and mechanical equipment. *Annals of Western Medicine and Surgery* 1950;**4**:687–716.
5. Wackers GL. Modern anaesthesiological principles for bulbar polio: manual IPPR in the 1952 polio-epidemic in Copenhagen. *Acta Anaesthesiologica Scandinavica* 1994;**38**:420–31.
6. Andersen EW, Ibsen B. The anaesthetic management of patients with poliomyelitis and respiratory paralysis. *British Medical Journal* 1954;**i**:786–8.
7. Kluger J. *Splendid Solution: Jonas Salk and the Conquest of Polio*. New York: Penguin, 2004.

Further reading

Gould T. *A Summer Plague. Polio and its Survivors*. New Haven and London: Yale University Press, 1995.

Paul JR. *A History of Poliomyelitis*. New Haven and London: Yale University Press, 1971.

13 From poliomyelitis to intensive care

On the 28 August 1953, a 16-year-old girl was admitted to the Ear, Nose and Throat Department of the Radcliffe Infirmary in Oxford with increasing respiratory paralysis and difficulty in swallowing. The doctors believed that the paralysis was caused by poliomyelitis. The patient was nursed in a tank ventilator in the prone position to allow the secretions to drain out of her mouth, but it became obvious that secretions were being sucked into the lungs and her condition was worsening. W Ritchie Russell and John Spalding, two Oxford neurologists who had visited Copenhagen shortly after the 1952 polio epidemic, decided that a tracheostomy should be performed and the patient ventilated with the prototype Radcliffe ventilator and humidification system that had recently been developed in Oxford (see Figure 9.5). A rota of doctors and nurses was organized to look after her throughout the 24 hours. Within a few days, she was completely paralysed, and only able to communicate by small movements of her eyes. At this point, a number of the other physicians questioned the ethics of keeping her alive.

Fortunately, it became apparent that the paralysis was due to acute toxic polyneuritis (otherwise known as Guillain–Barré syndrome), and not to poliomyelitis. The patient recovered and was discharged from hospital 6 weeks after she was admitted. She later became a nurse, worked in the respiration unit, married a farmer and had four children. Had the doctors looking after her decided that her case was hopeless, not only would she have died, but the adoption of this form of treatment would have been seriously delayed. Subsequently, other paralysed patients were treated in the Radcliffe Infirmary, although conditions were far from ideal. Finally, the Nuffield Hospitals Provincial Trust provided funding for a Respiration Unit at the Churchill Hospital in Oxford, and this was opened in 1955.[1]

Increasing use of intermittent positive-pressure ventilation

The girl whose life was saved at the Radcliffe Infirmary was one of the first in whom intermittent positive-pressure ventilation was used for a condition other than poliomyelitis. As has been described in Chapter 9, other workers were attempting to treat patients with severe tetanus by paralysing the muscles with curare and then providing artificial ventilation either with a tank ventilator or with manual compression of the bag in an anaesthetic breathing system, but treating such patients on the general hospital wards created an unsustainable load on the hospital staff. It was only when respiratory care units had been developed in the late 1950s that the prolonged use of intermittent positive-pressure ventilation became practicable.

After the establishment of such units, other successes were reported. In 1955, the Swedish surgeons Viking Olof Björk and Carl Gunnar Engström described how they had used the Engström ventilator to treat patients who were breathing inadequately after thoracic surgery,[2] and three years later one of the pioneers of Swedish anaesthesia, Olof Norlander, described how the technique had been used to treat other patients who had developed complications such as lung collapse or pneumonia after operation.[3]

One of the most dramatic uses of mechanical ventilation was reported in 1956. A 51-year-old Chicago railway worker was crushed and rolled into an 8-inch (20 cm) space between a train and a steel hearth furnace. To quote the authors' apt description of the accident '*Like pie-dough under a rolling pin his body diameter was reduced to the size of this space.*' The patient was moribund and in severe shock when admitted to hospital with multiple rib and other fractures, air in both pleural cavities, crush injuries to the liver and genitourinary tract, and paralysis of the gastrointestinal tract. Attempts were made to stabilize the chest by applying traction to pins inserted in the chest wall, but it was only when Trier Mørch* connected his piston ventilator to the cuffed tracheostomy tube that the patient's condition improved (Figure 13.1). The intermittent positive pressure from the ventilator inflated the lungs and so provided an internal splint for the ribs while the fractures healed. The patient remained on the ventilator for 30 days and left hospital 51 days later,

* E Trier Mørch was an innovative Copenhagen anaesthetist who was active in the Danish resistance movement during the Second World War. He was aware of Clarence Crafoord's use of a mechanical ventilator during thoracic surgery in Sweden in the late 1930s and constructed a piston ventilator from an iron water pipe during the war. He later emigrated to Chicago, where he promulgated the Danish techniques for treatment of respiratory failure.

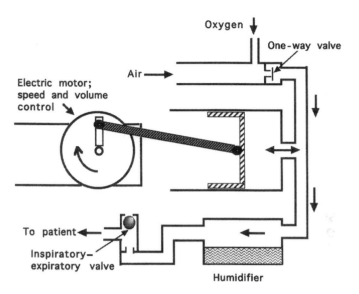

Figure 13.1 Trier Mørch's ingenious piston ventilator. The ventilator consisted of a simple piston pump with a table tennis ball valve that closed on inspiration and opened on expiration to allow the expired gas to flow to atmosphere. To save space, the ventilator was placed under the bed.

without any gross respiratory impairment. This incredible story revolutionized the treatment of crushing chest injuries.[4]

The origins of intensive care

There is no doubt that it was the experience gained in the 1952 Copenhagen poliomyelitis epidemic that led directly to the development of intensive care.[5] There were, however, four other important influences (Figure 13.2).

The first was the shock tent where the severely injured were resuscitated before being operated upon in the Second World War. By bringing these patients together, it was possible to provide a high level of monitoring and care.

The second was the introduction of units for the treatment of poisoning, which, in the 1950s, was predominantly due to the ingestion of barbiturate drugs.[6] The standard treatment of drug overdose had been to wash out the stomach and to give analeptic drugs that were supposed to diminish the duration of unconsciousness. This had limited success,

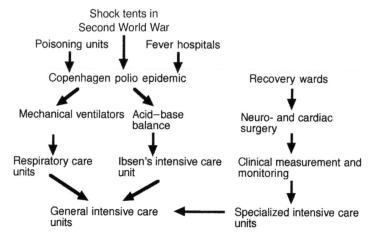

Figure 13.2 There were four major developments that ultimately led to the development of intensive care. The idea of concentrating patients requiring special care into dedicated units originated in the shock units of the Second World War, the poisoning units, the fever hospitals and the recovery rooms for postoperative patients. Mechanical ventilation and control of acid–base balance originated from the Copenhagen polio epidemic, while specialized monitoring emerged from the neurosurgical and cardiac recovery units.

but in 1950 the Swedish anaesthetist Eric Nilsson demonstrated that the most effective way to reduce mortality was to maintain a clear airway, to prevent the aspiration of secretions from the mouth into the lungs and to institute regular turning of the patient.[7] Nilsson's work led to the opening of a number of drug overdose units in Scandinavia and other European countries, but its real importance was that it showed that the application of routine anaesthetic techniques for looking after the unconscious patient could prevent the development of respiratory complications. This work provided the foundation for the nursing care now used in intensive care units.

The third factor that influenced the development of intensive care was the introduction of patient monitoring systems. When mechanical ventilation was first used to treat respiratory failure in the early 1950s, there were no rapid gas or blood gas analysers, and the few electrocardiographs remained firmly under the control of the cardiologists. Since there was no other monitoring equipment, the patient's condition was assessed by observation and clinical examination. The nursing staff recorded the usual measurements of temperature, pulse rate, blood pressure and fluid balance, and, if the patient was on a ventilator, they also recorded the airway pressure and expired volume to check that the machine was functioning correctly. By the end of the 1950s, mechanical ventilation was being used to treat patients suffering from a variety of causes of respiratory failure, including head injury, asthma, and acute-on-chronic bronchitis.[8] The doctors who were responsible for introducing mechanical ventilation into clinical practice soon realized that when the patient was sedated or paralysed, it was necessary to take responsibility for all of the body's functions that are normally controlled by the body's own control mechanisms. It therefore became routine practice to check the performance of each body system (central and peripheral nervous system, respiration, circulation, digestive system, kidney function, etc.) at frequent intervals during the day, and to take corrective action if abnormalities were found. It is the continual monitoring of all aspects of the patient's condition that characterizes intensive care today. The anaesthetist performs this function routinely in the operating theatre, so it was natural for anaesthetists to extend this practice to the recovery ward and then to the intensive care unit.

The fourth influence was the development of open-heart surgery in the early 1960s, for the measurement and monitoring techniques used in cardiac surgery were soon being utilized by those working in intensive care. By 1960, the first blood gas analysers for measuring oxygen and carbon dioxide levels and acid–base balance were becoming available, and electrocardiographs and electronic transducers for measuring blood pressures were being introduced into clinical practice. In the Hammersmith Hospital, doctors from other disciplines visiting the postoperative cardiac ward saw how monitoring was being used to guide therapy, and how mechanical ventilators were being used to provide respiratory support, and so started to refer acutely ill patients from their own wards. Thus the postoperative cardiac unit soon became a general intensive care unit. Units that initially only treated patients with acute respiratory failure were soon admitting patients with a wide range of acute life-threatening conditions, such as trauma, severe poisoning, and haemorrhagic or septicaemic shock. By the mid-1960s smaller four- to eight-bed intensive care units were being developed in district general hospitals, and during the next decade mechanical ventilation became a routine treatment for all types of severe respiratory failure, whether it was due to pneumonia, head injury, widespread sepsis, shock, heart failure or pulmonary oedema.[9,10]

Anaesthetists played a prominent role in all these initiatives, and in the UK over 80% of general intensive care units are still run by anaesthetists. The proportion is similar in most of the Scandinavian countries and in some other countries in Europe. In the USA, however, there has been a gradual decline in the number of anaesthetists running such units, most now being run by physicians or surgeons, many of whom have received part of their training in anesthesia departments, and have subsequently become accredited in the new speciality of critical care. A further difference between European and American practice is that whereas in Europe the doctors control all aspects of medical care and ventilator function, in the USA highly qualified respiratory therapists adjust and maintain the apparatus used for oxygen therapy and mechanical ventilation.[11,12]

Other types of unit: critical care

The benefits conferred by a dedicated intensive care unit were soon appreciated by other specialists. The cardiologists were among the first to develop specialized units for treating patients who had suffered a coronary thrombosis. Their requirements are, however, very different from those of the intensive care unit, for mechanical ventilation is rarely required, and the staff must be highly trained in the interpretation of the electrocardiograph, and skilled in dealing with cardiac emergencies. There are other specialized units such as neurosurgical units, burns units, and renal, heart, lung or liver transplant units. Premature baby units also began to add mechanical ventilation to their repertoire in the early 1960s, and were renamed special care units to mark their new role.

In recent years, there has been an increasing tendency to integrate intensive care and high-dependency care services and to relate them more closely to those provided by the accident and emergency department. This has resulted in the application of the American term 'critical care' to these services. In most parts of the UK, there are now emergency teams with doctors, nurses and paramedics, who are equipped and trained to provide medical assistance at any major disaster. There are a number of helicopter rescue services that are staffed by nurses, anaesthetists, and accident and emergency physicians, and many hospitals provide an anaesthetist to transport patients requiring intensive care from peripheral hospitals to major regional centres. Furthermore, much of the training of paramedics by anaesthetists and by accident and emergency doctors takes place in the operating theatre, intensive care unit, and accident and emergency department.

Problems in intensive care

The speciality of intensive care is concerned with acute medicine, with changes in the patient's condition taking place in seconds, minutes or hours rather than in days and months. Intensive care is concerned with the correction and treatment of organ malfunction, so that continuous monitoring of all of the body's functions is required. This is something that the anaesthetist does routinely in the operating theatre, and it is therefore logical that intensive care should be an integral part of the training of the anaesthetist. However, anaesthetists are involved in many other aspects of hospital activity, so it is not surprising that only a proportion of anaesthetists specialize in the intensive care field. Those who do so will have undertaken special training in medicine and in intensive care in addition to their five to six years of training as an anaesthetist. Similarly, physicians and surgeons who work in intensive care will have added a basic training in anaesthesia to their medical or surgical speciality training before taking up intensive care as a speciality. Nurses working in intensive care will also have undergone special training after their general four-year nursing training.

Working in an intensive care unit places special demands on all the staff, and especially on the nurses. The patients are seriously ill and require continuous attention. Most of the patients cannot speak, because of tracheal or tracheostomy tubes, but need constant encouragement and support. Mortality rates are inevitably in the region of 10–20% and there are many ethical problems to be faced. How do you explain to the relatives that the patient has irreversible brain damage? How do you ask them to give permission for organ donation? When and how do you switch off the ventilator when the patient is brain-dead? The combination of constant staff shortages, high workload and psychological stress creates a vicious circle that is difficult to break.

Despite these difficulties, intensive care is here to stay. The modern intensivist has to digest a vast amount of data generated by the many rapid analyses that can now be performed, and then has to modify therapy to ensure that all of the body's systems are performing optimally. The intensive care unit is a focus of activity for clinicians, nurses, radiologists, bacteriologists, clinical pathologists and many other supporting disciplines, and the therapeutic approach is distilled from the combined advice of many people. It is very different from the old approach where one consultant dictated treatment.

So, after 50 years, intensive care is still evolving. And, as we learnt in Chapter 12, all of this developed because the introduction of curare taught anaesthetists to control the ventilation, and because of that chance meeting between an infectious diseases doctor and an anaesthetist's wife while crossing the Atlantic in a large ocean liner.

References

1. Beinart J. *A History of the Nuffield Department of Anaesthetics, Oxford 1937–1987*. Oxford: Oxford University Press, 1987: 114.
2. Björk VO, Engström CG. The treatment of ventilatory insuffficiency after pulmonary resection with tracheostomy and prolonged artificial respiration. *Journal of Thoracic Surgery* 1955;**30**:356–67.
3. Norlander OP, Björk VO, Crafoord C, Friberg O, Hohlmdahl M, Swensson A, Widman B. Controlled ventilation in medical practice. *Anaesthesia* 1961;**16**:285–307.
4. Avery EE, Mörch ET, Benson DW. Critically crushed chests: a new method of treatment with continuous mechanical hyperventilation to produce alkalotic apnea and internal pneumatic stabilization. *Journal of Thoracic Surgery* 1956;**32**:291–311.
5. Ibsen B. Intensive therapy: background and development. *International Anesthesiology Clinics* 1966;**4**:277–94.
6. Clemmesen C. Treatment of acute barbituric acid poisoning. *International Anesthesiology Clinics* 1966;**4**:295–308.
7. Nilsson E. On treatment of barbiturate poisoning. *Acta Medica Scandinavica* 1951;**253** (Suppl):1.
8. Hilberman M. The evolution of intensive care units. *Critical Care Medicine* 1975;**3**:159–65.
9. Pearce DJ Experiences in a small respiratory unit of a general hospital. With special reference to the treatment of tetanus. *Anaesthesia* 1961;**16**:308–316.
10. Safar P, DeKornfeld TJ, Pearson JW, Redding JS. The intensive care unit. A three year experience in Baltimore City Hospitals. *Anaesthesia* 1961;**16**:275–84.
11. Groeger JS, Strosberg MA, Halpern NA, Raphaely RC, Kaye WE, Guntupalli KW et al. Descriptive analysis of critical care units in the United States. *Critical Care Medicine* 1992;**20**:846–63.
12. Hanson CW, Durbin CG, Maccioli GA, Deutschman CS, Sladen RN, Pronovost PJ, Gattinoni L. The anesthesiologist in critical care medicine. *Anesthesiology* 2001;**95**:781–8.

14 The tools of intensive care: mechanical ventilators and blood gas analysis

When the Copenhagen polio epidemic started, there were only three types of ventilator in common use. The first two – the tank ventilator (or 'iron lung') and the cuirass ventilator – expanded the lungs by producing an intermittent subatmospheric or 'negative' pressure around the chest wall. The third device – the rocking bed – utilized the weight of the abdominal viscera to move the diaphragm. Within a year of the end of the epidemic, manufacturers were focusing on the development of ventilators that inflated the lungs by applying intermittent positive pressure to the airway. Initially, these were simple mechanical pumps, but when microprocessors were introduced into medicine in the late 1970s, designers began to use pressurized gas sources and sophisticated valve control mechanisms to generate the pressures and flows required to ventilate the lungs. These ventilators are extremely versatile and can support ventilation in many different ways. As a result, a ventilator that cost a few hundred pounds in 1960 may now cost over £30 000.

'Negative-pressure' ventilators

Tank ventilator

Although there had been a number of attempts to develop a negative-pressure ventilator in the 19th century, it was not until 1929 that Philip Drinker and Louis Agassiz Shaw of Boston reported details of a tank ventilator that was suitable for clinical use.[1,2] The tank ventilator, colloquially known as the 'iron lung' (Figure 9.4), consisted of a large iron cylinder with several small ports that could be opened to provide nursing access. The patient lay on a mattress and frame that could be slid into the chamber from one end. The patient's head protruded through a tight and very uncomfortable rubber seal round the neck. The lungs could then be expanded by intermittently sucking the air out of the chamber with a large mechanically driven bellows, and expiration occurred when the chamber pressure was allowed to return to atmospheric.

Tank ventilators could be used successfully when paralysis was limited to the respiratory muscles, because such patients could close their larynx and swallow their pharyngeal secretions in synchrony with the ventilator. Unfortunately, there were many patients with a combined paralysis of the laryngeal, pharyngeal and respiratory muscles in the Copenhagen epidemic. In these patients, secretions were sucked into the lungs during inspiration and so produced collapse and infection in the lungs. This not only resulted in hypoxaemia but also made the lungs much stiffer than normal so it was difficult to inflate them with a tank or cuirass ventilator.

The Drinker type of ventilator was very expensive; it cost about $15 000 (the price of an average home at that time), but by 1931 a Boston engineer, Jack Emerson, had produced an improved model at half the cost. Many iron lungs were purchased in the USA with finance provided by charities such as 'The March of Dimes Fund', which encouraged the public to lay their dimes end-to-end on the pavement,[3] and, in American epidemics, it was not uncommon to see 30 or so of these tank ventilators working simultaneously in one large ward. It was an awesome sight and an extremely noisy environment for the patients and staff (Figure 12.2). In Britain, however, there were only 19 tank ventilators in the whole country in 1938.[4]

The Both ventilator

In the previous year, there had been a severe epidemic of poliomyelitis in South Australia, and an engineer named ET Both (Ted to his friends), ably assisted by his brother Donald, had designed and built a number of simple, cheap, fibreboard tank ventilators that functioned well in the clinical environment. Ted Both was a remarkable engineer, and had produced the first commercially available direct-writing electrocardiograph machine. In 1937, Both came to England to arrange for the manufacture of this machine under licence. While he was in London, another polio epidemic started. He offered his services to the London County Council, which was responsible for the fever hospitals where polio cases were treated, and started to manufacture his ventilators in North London (Figure 14.1).

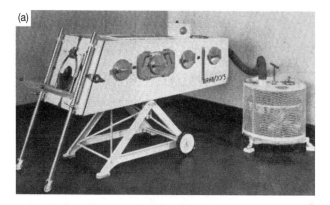

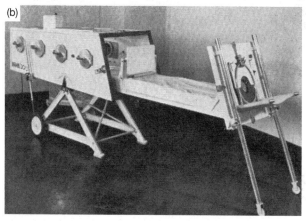

Figure 14.1 A Both Ventilator. This machine was developed by Ted Both in Australia and subsequently manufactured by Lord Nuffield in Oxford. It operated on the same principle as the Drinker ventilator, but was a much cheaper machine. The original design (see Figure 5.3) was modified in 1951 by GT Smith-Clarke, an engineer at the Alvis motor Company, and is here shown closed (a) and open (b). Smith-Clarke subsequently developed more sophisticated tank ventilators and intermittent positive-pressure ventilators. (Nuffield Department of Anaesthetics, Oxford.)

Robert Macintosh, who had just been appointed as the first Nuffield Professor in Anaesthetics at the University of Oxford, had been asked to deliver a lecture on artificial ventilation and decided to make a film showing the various methods that were available. He went to the Western Fever Hospital near London, where the Drinker and Both ventilators were being used, and there he met Ted Both. Shortly afterwards, Lord Nuffield was shown the film when he visited the Nuffield Institute for Medical Research in Oxford. Nuffield, who had founded the Morris Motor Company and had already made many medical benefactions (see Chapter 5), was advised by Macintosh that there was a widespread need for such a machine. On 23 November 1938, Nuffield announced that he would not only manufacture the Both machines at his car factory in Cowley, near Oxford, but would also donate one to every hospital in the British Commonwealth that requested one. By the end of 1939, 1600 Both ventilators had been allocated and some 800 actually delivered to hospitals in the UK and abroad, while training in their use was provided by members of the Nuffield Department of Anaesthetics in Oxford.[4]

Macintosh was a very innovative person, and in 1940 he reported that he had used a Both ventilator to support ventilation during the first 24 hours after operation in two patients who had undergone major surgery.[5] His idea was that the patient could be kept pain-free by administering large doses of opiate drugs, with the consequent respiratory depression being avoided by nursing them in the tank ventilator. As he later commented '*the practice was not continued because neither the surgeon nor the patient relished the idea of them waking up in a coffin*'.* Twenty years were to elapse before the introduction of intermittent positive-pressure ventilation to treat the postoperative respiratory depression caused by the analgesic drugs administered during anaesthesia for open-heart surgery.

Within a year of the Copenhagen epidemic, mechanical intermittent positive-pressure ventilators were being used for the treatment of bulbospinal poliomyelitis within the UK, but in the USA there was a delay in the development and use of such machines, and because of the widespread availability of tank ventilators, most patients were treated in these until the early 1960s. This resulted in an appreciable delay in the development of intensive care units in the USA.

Cuirass ventilator

The cuirass was a metal or plastic shell that was placed over the front of the chest and sealed to the body around the edge. Inspiration was produced by an electrically driven pump or large bellows that intermittently sucked the air out of the shell surrounding the chest, and so expanded the lungs. Expiration occurred when the pressure returned to atmospheric (see Figure 12.1). As Ibsen clearly demonstrated, the device was not very effective, but it could help to sustain ventilation when the patient was partially paralysed.

* Communication to the author.

The rocking bed

The bed was tilted rhythmically through about 45° by a mechanical rocking mechanism so that the weight of the abdominal contents raised and lowered the diaphragm. It was used to assist spontaneous respiration in patients with partial respiratory paralysis, but was relatively ineffectual and could only be used by those who were good sailors!

Intermittent positive-pressure ventilators

Two New York doctors, NW Green and HH Janeway, developed several intermittent positive-pressure mechanical ventilators that provided effective ventilation during thoracic surgery in animals during the period 1906–12. They not only kept a dog paralysed with curare alive for four hours, but also commented on the excellent operating conditions provided by the controlled ventilation.[6] Although Green went on to become a prominent thoracic surgeon, he never followed up his previous work in Janeway's laboratory, while Janeway changed direction and became a radiologist. It seems amazing that their answer to the problem of the open chest should be almost completely ignored for another 40 years.

Although several mechanical ventilators were developed during this time, there were few that proved effective in clinical practice. One that was used clinically was the Spiropulsator, which was developed by the Swedish ear, nose and throat surgeon P Frenckner and the engineer S Andersen. This was based on the flashing-light mechanism used in navigational buoys.[7] Although the Swedish surgeon Clarence Crafoord demonstrated how this ventilator could be used to provide controlled ventilation for thoracic surgery in the USA in 1940, it never became popular outside Sweden. E Trier Mørch, a most ingenious Danish anaesthetist, who, like a number of other Danish doctors, was an active member of the Resistance, had heard of the Spiropulsator and manufactured an electrically driven piston type of ventilator from an iron water pipe during the Second World War.[8] After the war, he moved to Chicago and built improved models with a one-way valve based on a table tennis ball. It was one of these machines that produced a dramatic recovery in a patient with a severe crushed chest injury (see Chapter 13 and Figure 13.1).

In the USA, two intermittent positive-pressure ventilators dominated the market in the postwar period. One was a flow-controlled ventilator that was designed by the aeronautical engineer RB Bennett. In this device, the inspiratory phase was triggered by the patient's inspiration, and the machine switched to expiration when the flow decreased at the end of inspiration. Since the machine breaths were synchronized with the patient's spontaneous respiration, the ventilator could be used to assist the breathing of a partially paralysed patient. A prototype of this machine was used successfully by Bower and his colleagues in the Los Angeles polio epidemic of 1948–49 to augment the ventilation of patients in a tank ventilator.[9,10] The other popular ventilator of the time was another patient-cycled machine designed by Forrest Bird of Palm Springs. He used it initially to nebulize bronchodilator drugs for treating asthma, but later it was used to provide respiratory support. Although it would seem logical to use ventilators that could be synchronized with the patient's breathing, there was a delay between the patient's inspiration and the machine's response, which made the ventilator inefficient in practice, and most American physicians remained wedded to the tank ventilator until the late 1950s.

The pioneer of ventilator development in the UK was JH Blease. He was an engineer who raced motorcycles and, as a sideline, had made some anaesthetic apparatus for a Liverpool anaesthetist before the Second World War. When the anaesthetist died, Blease found himself pressed into giving anaesthetics for casualties during the heavy air raids on Liverpool. Impressed by the drudgery of bag-squeezing during long thoracic operations, he designed and built a ventilator that could do the job. This was demonstrated at Wallasey Cottage Hospital in Liverpool in 1947. Although the production model appeared in 1950, it was several years before Blease ventilators became known in other centres.

In 1951, a Swedish surgeon, Carl Gunnar Engström, began to develop a much larger and very powerful piston type of ventilator that could both inflate the lungs with intermittent positive pressure and provide a subatmospheric (negative) pressure in the airways during expiration. At the time, it was believed that the negative pressure could offset some of the harmful effects of the positive pressure on the circulation. The Engström ventilator had one other advantage: it could use the opposite halves of the piston and cylinder to develop negative and positive pressures in a shell (or cuirass) that fitted tightly round the chest, so providing the motive power for both types of artificial ventilation. The Engström ventilator was tested on some of the patients at the end of the Danish epidemic and shown to be a very efficient machine, so the Swedish government immediately supported its further production. In the 1953 Swedish polio epidemic, all the patients with respiratory paralysis were successfully ventilated by these machines. The ventilator was subsequently marketed with great vigour, and, despite its high cost, was adopted widely throughout the world.[11]

Meanwhile, a number of other relatively simple machines were produced in Denmark, Germany, Sweden, France, and England.[12] The most successful machine in England was the Radcliffe ventilator developed by the neurologist Ritchie Russell and the engineer Edgar Shuster in Oxford in 1953.[13] The Radcliffe ventilator provided a mechanical drive for the Oxford inflating bellows, which had been developed for manual ventilation of the lungs (see Figure 9.5). The positive pressure was produced by weights on top of the bellows. The weighted bellows was expanded by an arm driven by an electric motor and then released, the respiration rate being adjusted by a two-speed clutch and a four-speed bicycle gearbox. These early ventilators were very primitive compared with present-day machines, but they proved to be reliable and were simple enough to be understood by those pioneering this form of treatment. They could also be maintained easily, and proved their worth in developing countries. There was, however, one major problem with both the Beaver and Radcliffe machines. Each used a simple non-rebreathing valve situated close to the patient to control the direction of gas flow in and out of the lungs. The valves were actuated by the pressures generated by the airflow, but tended to stick when wet. This was a lethal scenario that was later avoided by using cam-operated or electronic valves.

There was one other noteworthy contribution from Oxford, namely the 1953 development of a hot-water humidification system that ensured that secretions remained moist and so could be aspirated easily from the trachea.[14] Adequate humidification of the inspired gases is essential when the nose is bypassed, and the Oxford system provided optimal warming and moistening of the inspired gases with very simple equipment. Since blockage of the tracheostomy tube by dried secretions was an ever-present risk, this was probably one of the most important developments in respiratory care. More sophisticated versions of this system are now used routinely in intensive care units.

Most of the early ventilators were designed to impose a predetermined pattern of ventilation on the patient to ensure that ventilation was always adequate. During the past 20 years, it has become apparent that, in patients with stiff lungs, the resulting high airway pressures may produce further lung damage. Furthermore, there is now evidence that the distribution of gas within the lungs is improved if some spontaneous respiratory activity is maintained. In order to minimize these harmful effects, many new methods of assisting ventilation have been developed. As a result, the ventilators used today are much more sophisticated than previous machines, and they can provide many different patterns of controlled ventilation or assisted spontaneous ventilation.[15] Perfectly synchronized assistance to the patient's spontaneous breathing has only become possible because of the development of highly accurate flow sensors, pressure gauges and microprocessor control of very rapidly responding valves (Figure 14.2). Whether the increased cost and complexity of these new ventilators is justified by improved results has yet to be determined. Doctors are only human, however, and few of us would like to return to the Morris Cowley car or the Model T Ford.

Blood gas analysis

There was one other result of the Copenhagen polio epidemic that was important for the further development of medicine, namely the development of rapid methods of blood gas analysis. These enabled the clinician to determine the level of carbon dioxide and the acid–base status of the arterial blood, and so discover whether ventilation was adequate and whether there were other metabolic problems. The day after Ibsen had demonstrated how the clearance of secretions and manual ventilation of the lungs could return the 'total carbon dioxide in plasma' to normal levels, the clinical pathologist Poul Astrup borrowed a

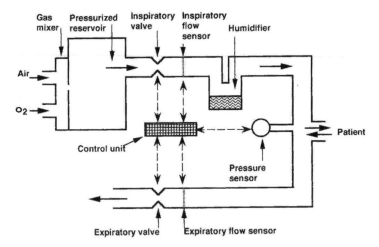

Figure 14.2 The design of a modern ventilator. Predetermined flows of compressed oxygen and air are delivered to the patient through rapidly acting computer-controlled valves. The resulting flow and pressure are sensed and the valves are servo-controlled to produce the desired flow or pressure waveform. Since the response of the valves is extremely rapid, the patient's spontaneous breathing can be assisted in many different ways.

prototype glass pH electrode and pH meter from a local firm called Radiometer, and confirmed that the blood from the patients with a high 'total carbon dioxide in plasma' was acid and not alkaline. As already mentioned in Chapter 12, this proved that the high level was due to decreased ventilation and not to kidney failure. Astrup realized that, even if he could measure the blood pH with the new electrode, he would still have problems in meeting the demand for blood gas analyses, because the measurement of 'total carbon dioxide in plasma' could only be made by skilled technicians, who took 20–30 minutes to analyse each blood sample on the Van Slyke apparatus.[16]

Astrup decided that a new approach was required, and over the next decade he and a close colleague, O Siggaard Andersen, cooperated with the Radiometer company to develop their new pH electrode. They then used this electrode to develop a revolutionary new interpolation technique for blood gas analysis. This enabled the acid–base status of the patient to be measured within a few minutes using three drops of blood. This was a tremendous advance, since the technique could be used on neonates as well as adults. Of even greater importance was the fact that Astrup and Siggaard Andersen introduced a new way of interpreting changes in acid–base balance that clarified the cause of the disturbance. The contributions of these workers revolutionized the understanding of the acid–base balance problems that are encountered in many disease states, and so enabled clinicians to apply the appropriate therapy without delay.[16]

While the Copenhagen workers were developing their technique, two workers in the USA were developing electrodes for measuring the oxygen and carbon dioxide levels in blood. One was Leland Clark, an electrochemist who developed an oxygen electrode for measuring gas or blood oxygen concentrations, and the second was John Severinghaus, an electronic engineer who later became a distinguished anaesthetist and respiratory physiologist. Severinghaus developed an electrode that provided direct measurements of carbon dioxide in gas and blood.[17] Oxygen and carbon dioxide electrodes are now combined with a pH electrode in automated systems that can print out the results of each analysis within a minute of injecting the blood sample. These tools enabled the anaesthetist to determine whether or not oxygenation and ventilation were adequate. However, of even more importance was the fact that we could begin to analyse the changes in lung function caused by various forms of lung disease. Anaesthetists were quick to adopt the new technology, and, in a number of hospitals, the anaesthetic department took over the responsibility for the analysis of the blood samples – yet another example of the growing influence of anaesthesia on the development of acute medicine. Now there are dedicated automated analysers that provide results within a minute or so in operating theatres and intensive care units throughout the hospital.

Over the last 50 years, advances in clinical measurement have revolutionized the care of the acutely ill patient because they enable the doctor to diagnose abnormalities in organ function and to follow the effects of therapy on a minute-to-minute basis. When we review the wide range of clinical measurements now available, we should remember that the initial impetus for their development sprang from the Copenhagen polio epidemic of 1952 and that their subsequent development has largely been driven by the needs of anaesthesia and intensive care.

References

1. Woollam CHM. The development of apparatus for intermittent negative pressure ventilation. (1) 1832–1918. *Anaesthesia* 1976;**31**:537–47.
2. Woollam CHM. The development of apparatus for intermittent negative pressure ventilation. (2) 1919–1976, with special reference to the development and uses of cuirass respirators. *Anaesthesia* 1976;**31**:666–685.
3. Gould T. *A Summer Plague. Polio and its Survivors*. New Haven and London: Yale University Press, 1995.
4. Macintosh RR. Mechanical respirators. *British Medical Journal* 1939;**ii**:83–6.
5. Macintosh RR. New use for the Both respirator. *Lancet* 1940;**ii**:745–6.
6. Green N, Janeway HH. Artificial respiration and intrathoracic oesophageal surgery. *Annals of Surgery* 1910;**52**:58–66.
7. Andersen E, Crafoord C, Frenckner P. A new and practical method of producing rhythmic ventilation during positive pressure anaesthesia. *Acta Otolaryngologica (Stockholm)* 1939;**28**:95–102.
8. Mørch ET. Controlled respiration by means of special automatic machines as used in Sweden and Denmark. *Anaesthesia* 1948;**3**:4–11.
9. Bower AG, Bennett VR, Dillon JB, Axelrod B. Investigation on the care and treatment of poliomyelitis patients. *Annals of Western Medicine and Surgery* 1950;**4**:561–82.
10. Bower AG, Bennett VR, Dillon JB, Axelrod B. Investigation on the care and treatment of poliomyelitis patients. Part 2. Physiological studies of various treatment procedures and mechanical equipment. *Annals of Western Medicine and Surgery* 1950;**4**:687–716.
11. Engström C-G. The clinical application or prolonged controlled ventilation. *Acta Anaesthesiologica Scandinavica* 1963; **Suppl XIII**.
12. Mushin WW, Rendell-Baker L, Thompson P, Mapleson WW. *Automatic Ventilation of the Lungs*, 2nd edn. Oxford: Blackwell Scientific, 1969.
13. Russell WR, Schuster E, Smith AC, Spalding JMK. Radcliffe respiration pumps. *Lancet* 1956;**i**:539–41.
14. Marshall J, Spalding JMK. Humidification in positive-pressure respiration for bulbospinal paralysis. *Lancet* 1953;**ii**:1022–4.

15. Sykes K, Young JD. *Respiratory Support in Intensive Care*. London: BMJ Books, 1999.
16. Astrup P, Severinghaus JW. *The History of Blood Gases, Acids and Bases*. Copenhagen: Munksgaard, 1986: 269–74.
17. Ibid: 280–91.

Further reading

Mørch ET. History of mechanical ventilation. In: Kirby RR, Banner MJ, Downs JB, eds. *Clinical Applications of Ventilatory Support*. London: Churchill Livingstone, 1990.
Sykes MK, Vickers MD, Hull CJ. *Principles of Measurement and Monitoring in Anaesthesia and Intensive Care*, 3rd edn. Oxford: Blackwell Scientific, 1991.

15 Anaesthesia for surgery on the heart

In 1893, the great German surgeon Theodore Billroth wrote '*Any surgeon who would attempt an operation on the heart should lose the respect of his colleagues*'. This remained the general view of most doctors for the next half-century. But once again it was experience gained in the Second World War that encouraged surgeons to rethink their attitude to this previously forbidden territory. In the immediate postwar period, surgeons started to dilate stenosed heart valves without opening the heart, but in the mid-1950s, hypothermia was being used to protect the brain while surgeons began to operate within the open heart. It was, however, the introduction of cardiopulmonary bypass that provided the opportunity for anaesthetists to take on a multidisciplinary role within the cardiac team. Some supervised the heart–lung machine, others were more interested in the problems of postoperative care, but all those involved with this type of surgery had to develop new techniques of anaesthesia, monitoring and clinical measurement. The techniques developed for cardiac surgery soon spread to other branches of anaesthesia and medicine, and so greatly improved the standard of care of the acutely ill patient.

The early days of heart surgery

There were two remarkable attempts to operate on the heart that preceded the main development by a quarter of a century. In 1923, Elliot Cutler in Boston introduced a knife through the wall of the left ventricle in a 12-year-old girl to split her stenosed mitral valve. She died, as did his next few patients, and he never attempted the operation again.[1] In England, on the 6 May 1925, Henry Souttar, a general surgeon, operated on a patient with mitral valve disease and managed to split the valve by inserting his finger into the valve through the left atrium. The anaesthetist was a surgeon, Mr Lindsay, and the patient was anaesthetized with ether that was blown down a narrow tube inserted into the trachea. Although the patient survived, Souttar's colleagues at the London Hospital were so shocked that he had dared to operate on the heart that they never referred another case.[2] But, as Bill Cleland, cardiac and thoracic surgeon, later commented, '*Perhaps this was just as well for disaster would surely have ensued, as with other attempts to attack the mitral valve in the 1920s. There was no blood transfusion service, no antibiotics and, perhaps most important, anaesthesia suitable for open chest surgery had not been developed*'.[3]

There were, however, two surgeons who were attempting to provide an alternative blood supply to the heart in patients who had disease of the coronary arteries. The first was Claude Beck, working in Cleveland, Ohio, and it was his work that aroused the interest of Leonard O'Shaughnessy, a surgeon who worked at Lambeth Hospital in London. In 1936, O'Shaughnessy began to graft intercostal muscles and omentum onto the heart muscle in an attempt to improve the blood supply. His anaesthetist, BK Hasler, writing in the *British Journal of Anaesthesia* in 1938/39, recorded that the Lambeth team had also dealt with patients with stab wounds or foreign bodies in the heart, and had even carried out the occasional pulmonary embolectomy. The anaesthetic technique was simple: a very heavy premedication, induction with ethyl chloride and maintenance with ether–oxygen delivered through a facemask. To maintain lung inflation in the open chest, positive pressure was applied by placing the opening from the expiratory tube under water.[4] Unfortunately, this work was terminated by O'Shaughnessy's death on the beaches of Dunkirk in 1940.

A new phase of cardiac surgery was initiated when the Boston paediatric surgeon RE Gross reported the successful closure of a patent ductus arteriosus in 1939. The cyclopropane anaesthesia was provided by Betty Lank, a nurse–anaesthetist.[5] Then, Helen Taussig, a specialist in children's heart problems at the John Hopkins Hospital in Baltimore, persuaded the newly appointed Professor of Surgery, Alfred Blalock, to join a branch of the aorta to the pulmonary artery so that some of the desaturated blood leaving the heart in children with congenital heart disease could be rerouted through the lungs. Blalock had established his reputation at Vanderbilt University Medical School with fundamental research on the causes of surgical shock. He had been assisted by a highly skilled black technical assistant, Vivien Thomas. The two had a great respect for each other, and when Blalock moved to Baltimore in 1941, he brought Thomas with him.* In 1943, Blalock and Thomas embarked on a series of animal experiments to develop the techniques required for the new type of surgery, and on 29 November 1944, as Allied troops marched across Europe, Merel Harmel and Austin Lamont anaesthetized the 15-month-old 'blue baby' who had been selected for the operation.[6] Because most anaesthetists were heavily involved in routine anaesthesia, it was not common for them to participate in an experimental surgical programme, so Harmel and Lamont had little idea how the baby might respond to the anaesthesia and surgical procedure. Fortunately, the infant survived, and Blalock went on to perform a further 200 similar procedures. In 1946, Harmel and Lamont described the problems in anaesthetizing these extremely ill children, but were able to report a survival rate of nearly 80%.[7]

Towards the end of the war, an American surgeon, Dwight Harken, who had received part of his training at the Brompton Hospital for Diseases of the Chest in London, returned to Britain as Chief Surgeon at the American Surgical Chest Center in Cirencester. Harken began to remove bullets and shrapnel from the heart, and in 1946 reported that he had operated on 134 cases, 56 of whom had objects closely related to the heart or great vessels, and 13 of which were actually within the heart cavity or a blood vessel. Incredibly, none of these patients died.[8] This demonstrated once and for all that the heart was a very robust organ that could withstand handling and surgery.

Another phase of cardiac surgery began in 1948 when surgeons began to operate blindly within the heart using a finger or mechanical dilator to split open narrowed mitral or pulmonary valves – the phase of 'closed' cardiac surgery.[9] The third phase – 'open-heart' surgery – began in 1953 when surgeons began to operate on the inside of the heart under direct vision. They could do so only if the heart contained no blood. Since the empty heart could not eject blood into the aorta, it was necessary either to protect the body tissues from a lack of oxygen by cooling (induced hypothermia) or to feed an artificial supply of oxygenated blood into the aorta from an extracorporeal circuit containing a heart–lung machine.

---

* Although Thomas directed Blalock's research laboratories and taught many young surgeons, he encountered racial prejudice and segregation both in Baltimore city and in the hospital. He was not allowed to eat in the same cafeteria as Blalock, and had to moonlight as a bartender to support his family. When Blalock died in 1965, Thomas suffered severe depression for six years, but in the 1970s, as desegregation crept into the hospital, Thomas's contribution was recognized and he was awarded an honorary doctorate. He died in 1985 at the age of 75.

Open-heart surgery

Induced hypothermia

It was in 1950 that WG Bigelow and his colleagues in Toronto first demonstrated that a reduction in body temperature could protect body tissues during a brief arrest of the circulation. They showed in animals that a reduction in body temperature from 37°C to 30°C could prolong the period that the brain could tolerate the lack of a blood supply from 3 minutes to 8–10 minutes.[10] In 1953, FW Lewis in Minneapolis became the first surgeon to close an atrial septal defect by inducing hypothermia with cooling blankets, but most other surgeons subsequently used a technique developed by Henry Swan in Denver; this involved cooling the patient in a bath of iced water.[11] The surgeon Holmes Sellors and the anaesthetist Brian Sellick used this technique extensively at the Middlesex Hospital in London, and in 1960 reported a series of 200 cases operated on in this manner.[12]

It was, however, a rather cumbersome and wet procedure.[13] After attaching the monitoring apparatus, the patient was anaesthetized and intubated (curare being given to prevent shivering), and then lifted into the bath with all the monitoring leads and intravenous infusions attached. Buckets of ice were added to the bath water, which was then stirred vigorously with wooden spoons. The temperature in the oesophagus was carefully monitored, and the patient was lifted onto the operating table when it reached 32°C. This allowed for the continued fall in temperature that occurred while the surgeon was opening the chest. There was then an extremely tense few minutes while the surgeon tightened snares around the great veins, opened the heart, examined the defect, attempted to repair it, refilled the heart with blood, tried to eliminate all the air bubbles, and then restarted the heartbeat by electrical defibrillation. When the operation was over, the patient had to be rewarmed in a similar fashion. This brought the total time for the procedure to about 6 hours. For this reason, Russell Brock at the Brompton Hospital developed a system that cooled and warmed the patient's blood by circulating it through a heat-exchanging device. This was a neater but technically more complicated system, and the patient had to receive anticoagulant drugs to prevent blood from clotting in the circuit.

But the most serious problem of any technique using cooling to 30°C was that the time for operating within the heart was limited to 6–8 minutes. If the defect turned out to be more complicated than expected, the surgeon had only two choices: he had to either leave the repair incomplete or risk leaving the patient with severe brain damage. It was this dilemma that added further impetus to the development of extracorporeal circulation with the use of the heart–lung machine.

Extracorporeal circulation

The principle of extracorporeal circulation is simple (Figure 15.1). After the chest has been opened and the heart exposed, two large cannulae are inserted into the superior and inferior venae cavae. Another cannula is situated in a large peripheral artery or in the aorta close to the heart. The heart–lung machine is primed with fluid, and all visible air bubbles are removed from the circuit. The venous blood returning to the heart is

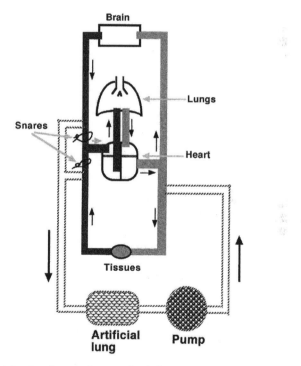

Figure 15.1 Cardiopulmonary bypass circuit. Large cannulae are inserted into the superior and inferior venae cavae so that all the venous return is directed to the bypass circuit when the snares are tightened. Another cannula is inserted into the aorta near to the heart. Blood drains from the venae cavae into the oygenator and is then pumped back into the aorta. The oxygenated blood circulates around the body and is drained back into the heart–lung machine.

gradually diverted into the artificial lung by tightening two snares around the cannulae in the venae cavae. Meanwhile, the arterial pump is gradually brought up to speed so that it pumps a similar amount of blood from the artificial lung back into the aorta. The machine operator has to achieve a delicate balance between the amount of blood entering and leaving the machine to ensure that the volume of blood in the patient is unchanged. The operator has two other responsibilities: control of the flow and composition of the gas passing through the artificial lung (to ensure that the oxygen and carbon dioxide levels and pH are held within the normal range) and control of blood temperature (which is usually reduced to about 30°C to help protect the brain during bypass).

When bypass has been established, the only blood entering the heart is from the coronary arteries. This blood provides nutrients and oxygen to the heart muscle, and drains to the inside of the heart, where it is removed by a suction catheter and returned to the machine. Thus the heart can be opened and the lesion can be corrected under direct vision, bypass times usually varying from a half to two, three or even four hours.

The procedure sounds simple, but it took John Gibbon and his wife nearly 20 years to solve all of the technical problems involved.[14] They had to learn to cannulate major blood vessels without spilling blood; they had to create an artificial lung that could replace the tennis court-sized surface area of the human alveolae; they had to develop safe methods of preventing blood clotting; and they had to pump the blood around the circuit without damaging the red cells. They started work on the development of a heart–lung machine in Boston in 1934, and finally, in 1952, Gibbon operated on his first human case at the Jefferson Medical College in Philadelphia, where he had become Professor of Surgery. The patient was a 15-month-old baby who turned out to have a more complicated defect than the simple hole in the atrial septum that had been expected. She died. In 1953, Gibbon operated on an 18-year-old girl who survived, but his next two operations resulted in death. Gibbon was so devastated that he vowed never to undertake cardiac surgery again. Although he was only 53 years old and at the height of his powers, Gibbon never published another paper.

The development of open-heart surgery at the Hammersmith Hospital

Developments in Europe were not far behind. In Sweden, the surgeon Viking Olof Björk had produced a rotating-disc oxygenator in the late 1940s.[15] Dennis Melrose, a surgical research worker at the Postgraduate Medical School, London, had seen this machine and constructed an improved version that was tested at the Royal Veterinary College in

London (Figure 15.2). In 1953, the surgeon Bill Cleland, Melrose and the team at the Hammersmith Hospital in London decided to use the machine to provide partial circulatory support during closed surgery for valve disease.[16,17] The first two patients survived, but the next four died, so further clinical work was stopped. In 1956, Melrose and Cleland paid lengthy visits to John Kirklin at the Mayo Clinic, Rochester and C Walton Lillehei in Minneapolis, where they learnt of the vital importance of monitoring, and the maintenance of fluid and blood balance. They put this experience to the test on 17 April 1957 by successfully closing an atrial septal defect, but there was still a great deal of scepticism from their colleagues. With the support of Richard Bonham Carter, paediatric cardiologist at the Hospital for Sick Children, Great Ormond Street, London, they took the bold decision to operate on a series of 50 children with ventricular septal defects, with no questions

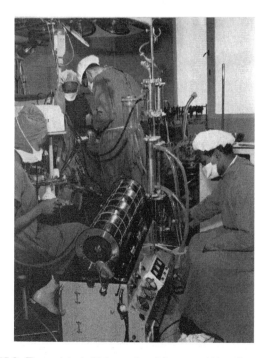

Figure 15.2 The original Melrose heart–lung machine in use at the Hammersmith Hospital, London in 1961. The oxygenator is the large rotating cylinder on the top of the machine.

being asked about progress until the trial was completed. This was a time of immense stress for the members of the team, since an operation provided the only hope for most of these terminally ill children. In the event, the trial was a resounding success. Although there was an overall mortality rate of 20%, because only the sickest children were selected for operation, the mortality rate was only 4% in uncomplicated cases.[18] This established the technique once and for all in the UK.

The problems for the anaesthetist

The major problem in the early days of open-heart surgery was that most of the patients had advanced cardiac disease, so the risk of anaesthesia and surgery was high.[19] Patients and their relatives knew the risk they were taking, but they also realized that there was no alternative. Those with congenital abnormalities of the heart were often young and frightened by the idea of an operation, and there were the additional technical problems of cannulating tiny arteries and veins. So what was different about anaesthesia for open-heart surgery?

First, there was the premedication. Although every care was taken to explain the procedure at the preoperative visit, patients were naturally very frightened. To ensure a good night's sleep, they received a barbiturate on the night before operation and another dose in the morning. The anaesthetist then visited the patient an hour before surgery and prescribed additional premedication so that they were well sedated when they came to theatre.

The second difference was that it took much longer to prepare the patient for operation. At that time, the only monitoring used during routine anaesthesia was clinical observation of the skin colour and the rate and depth of breathing, a finger on the pulse, and a sphygmomanometer cuff around the arm. Monitoring the patient undergoing open-heart surgery, however, was an altogether more complex affair. After checking their identity label, notes and X-rays, the patient was transferred to the operating table, which had been moved into the anaesthetic room. The blood pressure cuff and electrocardiograph leads were attached, and one or two intravenous cannulae were inserted for drug injections and blood transfusion. A metal (later plastic) cannula was inserted into the radial artery for more accurate blood pressure measurement and blood sampling, and a long catheter was passed into one of the great veins so that central venous pressure could be used as a guide to transfusion. (Later, venous pressure was measured through a catheter inserted into the internal jugular vein in the neck, a procedure requiring even greater technical skill.) After these preparations, anaesthesia was induced very slowly and carefully, a tracheal tube was inserted, temperature-measuring probes were inserted into the oesophagus and rectum, the diathermy earth lead was attached, and a catheter was inserted into the bladder to measure urine output. Finally, the operating table, together with the electrocardiograph, drip stands and the anaesthesia machine/ventilator were wheeled into the operating theatre. The whole procedure took about 30 minutes if everything went well. If it didn't, the surgeon had to sip another cup of coffee.

In the theatre, the arterial and venous pressure lines were connected to the pressure transducers, and the pressure traces and electrocardiograph were displayed on a large oscilloscope screen that could be seen by all the team (Figure 15.3). There were also large dials that could be seen by the heart–lung machine operator. The mechanical ventilator was set to deliver an appropriate volume of anaesthetic gas mixture, and the airway

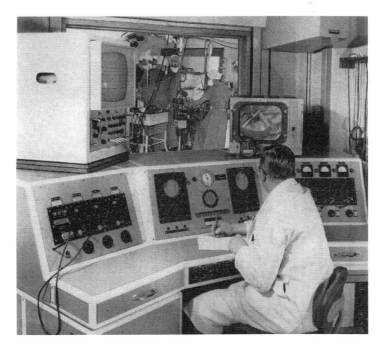

Figure 15.3 View of recording room with operating theatre in the background at the Hammersmith Hospital, London in 1961. To the left is the oscilloscope that displayed the arterial pressure waveform and electrocardiograph, and to the right is the closed-circuit television that displayed the surgical field.

pressure and expired gas volume were monitored by a pressure gauge and gas meter on the machine. Blood gas and potassium measurements were taken at intervals before, during and after bypass, and clotting tests were performed at regular intervals. Blood loss was estimated by weighing swabs and measuring loss in the suction reservoir, and urine flow was measured in another container. All of these measurements had to be charted at regular intervals. For several years, we also measured brain activity with an electroencephalograph (Figure 15.4). In short, everything that could be monitored was, and all the drugs used to control blood pressure or correct cardiac irregularities were close at hand.[20]

This was a much more complex scenario than the anaesthetist had been used to, so those embarking on this kind of project had a lot to learn. He or she not only had to develop new technical skills, but also had to acquire an in-depth knowledge of cardiovascular, respiratory and renal physiology so that the measurements could be correctly interpreted and the appropriate therapy instituted. Because the mechanical ventilator took over ventilation, and the heart–lung machine replaced both the heart

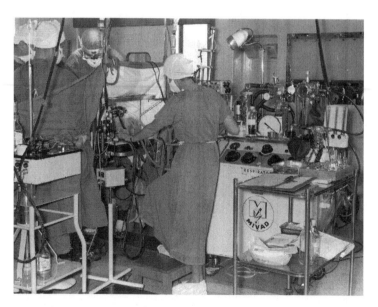

Figure 15.4 Anaesthesia for open-heart surgery at the Hammersmith Hospital, London in 1961. The Engström ventilator is to the right of the anaesthetist, and the equipment for measuring arterial and venous pressures is on the small table to the left.

and the lungs during bypass, the anaesthetist had an exceptional opportunity to learn how each component affected the functioning of the whole body. This was very different from the simple manual control of ventilation that had recently been adopted for thoracic surgery.

Cardiopulmonary bypass

During bypass, the exchange of gas and the circulation of the blood were under the control of the pump operator, so the anaesthetists could take it in turn to slip out for a quick coffee. At the end of bypass, there was a lot of activity as the surgeon restarted the heart. The electrical defibrillator had to be charged and discharged, calcium or other cardiac drugs injected to stimulate the heart contractions or treat irregularities, and protamine injected to reverse the action of the anticoagulant drug. The next two or three hours were spent transfusing blood into the circulation while the surgeons attempted to seal all the bleeding points and close the chest. Six to seven litres of blood were routinely used for each case. In the 1960s, most of the patients were on the operating table for 6–8 hours, and it was not uncommon to have to reopen the chest later that night to deal with postoperative bleeding. Fortunately, the whole procedure is now accomplished within a few hours, and it is not uncommon for one team to perform several bypass operations in one day. It is even more remarkable that blood transfusion may not be required.

The postoperative period

In the Hammersmith Hospital, the patients who had undergone open-heart surgery were initially nursed in small side-rooms off the general wards, but these could not accommodate our ventilators or other equipment. In 1961, our surgical team managed to persuade the hospital authorities to build a seven-bed postoperative recovery area close to the operating theatres, and this soon became a centre of activity. By now, our anaesthetic department research technicians were providing a blood gas analysis service using Poul Astrup's system, and we were able to make a series of measurements that showed that patients who had undergone open-heart surgery had an abnormality of lung function that we called 'post-perfusion lung'.[21] These patients not only suffered from the usual postoperative pulmonary complications, but also had an additional problem that seriously affected the transfer of oxygen across the lungs. At that time, we had no idea what was causing the problem, but it is now known that this is an immunological response to the blood used to prime the pump before bypass.

It soon became obvious that patients might develop respiratory failure at any time during the first few days after operation.[22] They needed continuous monitoring of circulation, respiration and kidney function, and the only way to achieve this was to provide what has now become known as intensive care. We watched the patients' progress very carefully. If they developed cardiac or respiratory failure, we would anaesthetize them, insert a tracheal tube, and connect them to a mechanical ventilator. With this technique, we could ensure that blood gases were returned to normal levels, and this, in itself, often helped the cardiac condition. Fortunately, the first three cases we treated with this technique survived, although one patient had three successive cardiac arrests that were treated successfully while she was on the ventilator. She subsequently returned to her Somerset village and had four children. As the benefits of postoperative mechanical ventilation became apparent, we began to transfer patients who were in poor condition at the end of the operation to a ventilator in the intensive care unit without attempting to re-establish consciousness and spontaneous ventilation.[23]

And so to intensive care

Success with the open-heart surgery patients brought us other postoperative patients with respiratory failure, and soon patients with tetanus and other conditions were referred from the medical wards. Thus, from our beginnings as a postoperative recovery ward for open-heart surgery patients, we became a general intensive care unit.

It must be emphasized that when we started this unit, we still knew very little about the effects of mechanical ventilation on the function of the lung or on the circulation. Thanks to the early pioneers in the polio units, we had learnt the basics of respiratory care, but we then had to train nurses and physiotherapists to carry out this highly specialized care for many different kinds of patient. It was fortunate that we had been able to get research funding that enabled us to acquire an Astrup apparatus for blood gas measurement, together with equipment for measuring arterial blood pressure and cardiac output, so we could begin to analyse cardiac and respiratory function during and after operation. With these facilities, we were able to define which patients were likely to benefit from our ministrations and so help our surgical colleagues cope with some of the complex problems with which they were presented. By the late 1960s, intensive care units were being opened in many other hospitals, and now every anaesthetist receives special training in intensive care.

But perhaps the most important benefit that anaesthetists gained from participation in the open-heart surgery programme was the increased understanding of the circulation and the advantages to be gained from invasive monitoring. For example, at the end of bypass, the pump operator uses the venous pressure as a guide to the volume of blood that should be left in the patient, and the anaesthetist continues to use this measurement to guide blood replacement in the postoperative period. The value of venous pressure measurement was described in 1963, and within a short time it became the standard technique for assessing the adequacy of transfusion in the UK.[24] There were many other developments that were eventually incorporated into general anaesthetic practice.

Cardiac surgery today

In the early days of open-heart surgery, most of the operations were for the correction of congenital abnormalities. In the 1960s, surgeons began to repair damaged valves by inserting either a homograft or an artificial valve. In the 1970s, coronary arterial bypass grafts moved into the ascendancy, while a few units started to transplant the heart. Now, bypass grafts constitute about 90% of the work of cardiac surgery units. Most units continue to use extracorporeal circulation for these procedures, but in some the grafts are inserted while the heart is still beating, thus avoiding the disadvantages associated with cardiopulmonary bypass. Minimally invasive surgical techniques are being increasingly used.

There was one other anaesthetic contribution that arose directly out of the anaesthetist's involvement with cardiac surgery, namely the development of resuscitation services outside the operating theatre environment. As we shall see in the next chapter, this is a story that takes us back to biblical times.

References

1. Cutler EC, Levine SA. Cardiotomy and valvulotomy for mitral stenosis. *Boston Medical and Surgical Journal* 1923;**188**:1023–7.
2. Ellis RH. The first trans-auricular mitral valvotomy. *Anaesthesia* 1975;**30**:374–90.
3. Cleland WP. The evolution of cardiac surgery in the United Kingdom. *Thorax* 1983;**38**:887–96.
4. Hasler JK. Anaesthesia in cardiac surgery. *British Journal of Anaesthesia* 1938/39;**16**:30–4.
5. Gross RE, Hubbard JP. Surgical ligation of patent ductus arteriosus: report of first successful case. *Journal of the American Medical Association* 1939;**112**:729–31.
6. Blalock A, Taussig HB. Surgical treatment of malformations of heart in which there is pulmonary stenosis or pulmonary atresia. *Journal of the American Medical Association* 1945;**128**:189–202.
7. Harmel MH, Lamont A. Anesthesia in the surgical treatment of congenital pulmonic stenosis: preliminary report. *Anesthesiology* 1946;**7**:477–98.
8. Harken DE. Foreign bodies in, and in relation to, thoracic blood vessels and

heart. 1 – Techniques for approaching and removing foreign bodies from chambers of heart. *Surgery, Gynecology and Obstetrics* 1946;**83**:117–25.

9. Historical session 1. The emergence of cardiac surgery. *Journal of Thoracic and Cardiovascular Surgery* 1989;**98**:805–51.

10. Bigelow WG, Lindsay WK, Greenwood WF. Hypothermia: its possible role in cardiac surgery. An investigation of factors governing survival in dogs at low body temperatures. *Annals of Surgery* 1950;**132**:849–66.

11. Swan H, Zeavin I, Holmes JH, Montgomery V. Cessation of circulation in general hypothermia: physiologic changes and their control. *Annals of Surgery* 1953;**138**:360–76.

12. Bedford DE, Holmes Sellors T, Somerville W, Belcher JR, Besterman EMM. Atrial septal defect and its surgical treatment. *Lancet* 1957;**ii**:1255–71.

13. Sellick BA. A method of hypothermia for open heart surgery. *Lancet* 1957;**ii**:443–6.

14. LeFanu J. *The Rise and Fall of Modern Medicine*. London: Little Brown, 1995.

15. Björk VO. Brain perfusions in dogs with artificially oxygenated blood. *Acta Chirurgica Scandinavica*. 1948;**96**(Suppl 137):1–122.

16. Melrose DG, Aird I. A mechanical heart–lung for use in man. *British Medical Journal* 1953;**ii**:57–62.

17. Aird I, Melrose DG, Cleland W, Lynn RB. Assisted circulation by pump–oxygenator during operative dilatation of the aortic valve in man. *British Medical Journal* 1954;**i**:1284–7.

18. Cleland WP, Beard AJ, Bentall HH et al. The treatment of ventricular septal defect. *British Medical Journal* 1958;**ii**:1369–77.

19. Beard A.JW. The anaesthetic management of patients for extracorporeal circulation. *Proceedings of the Royal Society of Medicine* 1958;**51**:598–91.

20. Sykes MK. The role of the anaesthetist in extracorporeal circulation. *Proceedings of the Royal Society of Medicine* 1962;**55**:187–94.

21. McClenahan JB, Young WE, Sykes MK. Respiratory changes after open-heart surgery. *Thorax* 1965;**20**:545–54.

22. Gilston A. The management of respiratory distress after cardiothoracic surgery. *Thorax* 1962;**17**:139–45.

23. Sandison JW, McCormick PW, Sykes MK. Intermittent positive pressure respiration after open-heart surgery. *British Journal of Anaesthesia* 1963;**35**:100–13.

24. Sykes MK. Venous pressure as a clinical indicator of adequacy of transfusion. *Annals of the Royal College of Surgeons of England* 1963;**33**:185–97.

Further reading

Hurt R. *The History of Cardiothoracic Surgery from Early Times*. Carnforth: Parthenon, 1996.

Norlander O, Pitzele S, Edling I, Norberg B, Crafoord C, Senning A. Anesthesiological experience from intracardiac surgery with the Crafoord–Senning heart–lung machine. *Acta Anaesthesiologica Scandinavica* 1958;**2**:181–210.

Norlander O, Björk VO, Crafoord C, Friberg O, Holmdahl M, Swensson A, Widman B. Controlled ventilation in medical practice. *Anaesthesia* 1961;**16**:285–307.

Spencer FC, Benson DW, Liu WC, Bahnson HT. Use of a mechanical respirator in the management of respiratory insufficiency following trauma or operation for cardiac or pulmonary disease. *Journal of Thoracic and Cardiovascular Surgery* 1959;**38**:758–79.

Westaby S. *Landmarks in Cardiac Surgery*. Oxford: Isis Medical Media, 1997.

16 Resuscitation of the apparently dead

I (KS) was in a rear aisle seat and sitting next to a quiet Norwegian businessman as the small plane twisted and turned to land at Oslo airport in 1961. I saw my neighbour's head suddenly fall forwards. His skin was pale and sweaty, he was not breathing, and he did not respond when I grabbed his wrist to feel his pulse. There was no pulse and his pupils were widely dilated. I was going to Oslo to attend a meeting on resuscitation, so what could I do but start the emergency drill for the treatment of cardiac arrest?

There followed one of those situations where farce and tragedy are inextricably intertwined. I realized that I could do nothing while the victim was in his seat, and that if I delayed treatment until we landed it would be too late. So I rang the bell for the steward, undid the seat belts and tried to haul my neighbour's body into the narrow gangway. The steward arrived and insisted that we both get back into our seats. I told him I was a doctor and the patient needed treatment for a cardiac arrest. The turbulence became worse and the steward retreated to his seat. After much heaving and cursing, I managed to drag the body into the aisle and to start mouth-to-mouth ventilation and cardiac compression. To my surprise and delight, the patient started to breathe and, as we touched down, he started to recover consciousness.

He later told me that he suffered from an ear problem that sometimes produced severe pain during descent from altitude, and that this had caused him to become unconscious once before. Presumably he had suffered reflex slowing of the heart as a result of the acute pain in his ear, and the resulting decrease in blood supply to the brain had caused the loss of consciousness and dilatation of the pupils. Probably, his tongue then fell back and obstructed his airway so that he could not breathe, and I failed to detect a pulse because of the vibration of the engines. It was a happy misdiagnosis on my part, but if I had failed to take action he might have developed a true cardiac arrest and never recovered. As I left the plane, the steward again reprimanded me for endangering the lives of all on board by leaving my seat.

The ABC of resuscitation

The techniques used for resuscitating the airline passenger are known as the ABC of resuscitation, with the initials standing for the sequence 'Airway, Breathing and Circulation'. Mouth-to-mouth resuscitation was mentioned in the Bible (2 Kings 4, vv.34–5), so it might be assumed that it had been the standard treatment for hundreds of years. In fact, the ABC of resuscitation was not introduced until the 1960s, and even then it was difficult to persuade official bodies that it should supplant the older methods. Since anaesthetists were responsible for the reintroduction of mouth-to-mouth ventilation, and now play a major role in the organization of resuscitation services, we should ask why it took so long for this apparently simple technique to be reinstated.

Resuscitation in bygone times

The possibility of restoring life after apparent death has fascinated man since the earliest times, but although mouth-to-mouth breathing may have been practised by the ancient Egyptians and is mentioned in the Bible, in the ensuing years it was mainly used by midwives attempting to resuscitate newborn babies.[1] It may seem surprising that air that has been expired from the lungs of the rescuer should be able to supply enough oxygen to the victim. The explanation is simple: the first 150 ml of air that enters the victim's lungs comes from the airways of the rescuer and so has neither given up oxygen nor gained carbon dioxide. The remainder of the breath comes from the operator's alveoli, but contains plenty of oxygen, since the operator tends to breathe more deeply than normal.

Mouth-to-mouth resuscitation

The first record of a successful mouth-to-mouth resuscitation in an adult appears to have been that carried out by William Trossack in 1732, but it was only when this was reported to the Royal Society in 1756 that scientists began to take an interest in the whole subject of resuscitation.[2]

Possibly because of the conjunction between the large number of canals in the Netherlands and the enjoyment of alcohol, the Dutch had always taken an interest in resuscitation, and in 1767 they created a society whose aim was to reduce the mortality from drowning. Their recommended regime included warming the patient, mouth-to-mouth respiration, the introduction of tobacco smoke into the rectum (a well-known stimulant) and vigorous rubbing of the patient. Within 25 years of its formation, the society had accumulated reports of over 990 successful resuscitations. The success of the Dutch organization stimulated the formation of a similar society in London in 1774; this subsequently became the Royal Humane Society. The famous surgeon of the day, John Hunter, became interested in the problem and investigated the use of a bellows to provide the artificial ventilation.[3]

The Royal Humane Society supported the use of a bellows to blow air into the lungs (Figure 16.1), but the difficulty was to provide an airtight connection between the bellows and the airway. Although there were tubes that could be guided into the larynx by the fingers, few people could carry out this difficult manoeuvre, and the alternative tubes, designed to be plugged into the nostrils, were not so effective because the air leaked out through the mouth.[4] Nevertheless, successful resuscitations were reported over the next half-century. Then, in 1827/28, a French surgeon, J Leroy, published experimental work showing that overenthusiastic use of the bellows could rupture the lungs of the victim.[5] Endorsement of this work by the French Academy of Sciences resulted in the abandonment of resuscitation by bellows. At the same time, scientists

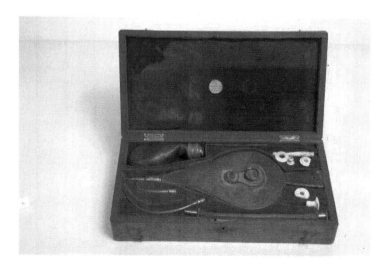

Figure 16.1 Royal Humane Society Resuscitation box containing bellows and nasal and oral tubes – late 18th century. (Nuffield Department of Anaesthetics, Oxford.)

who were beginning to understand the nature of gases began to question whether the gas expired from the lungs was suitable for resuscitation. The result was that the use of mouth-to-mouth ventilation declined and doctors began to develop other methods of artificial respiration.

Manual methods

The manual methods of artificial ventilation that were developed in the 19th century were designed to move air in and out of the lungs by altering the stresses on the chest wall. The advantage claimed for such a technique was that it required no apparatus and so could be used in almost any situation by anyone who had been trained in first-aid. The first technique, which involved hip lifting and chest compression, was described by a general practitioner, Marshall Hall, in 1856. In 1858, another practitioner, HR Silvester, described the arm-lift chest pressure method. The Shäfer prone chest-pressure method followed in 1902, and the Holger Nielsen prone back-pressure arm-lift method and the Eve rocking method in 1932.

A few years later, the anaesthetists Ralph M Waters and James H Bennett in Madison, Wisconsin, reviewed the literature and found that over 70 manual methods had been described. There were, however, no studies to show whether these methods were effective. In 1936, they reported that they had made measurements on unconscious, intubated patients who had been rendered apnoeic by hyperventilation during ether anaesthesia. They found that the Sylvester technique produced the largest breaths, but they realized that, when the patient was unconscious but not intubated, the airway might become obstructed since the Sylvester technique could only be performed with the patient lying on the back.[6]

In 1941, a junior anaesthetist in the Nuffield Department of Anaesthetics at Oxford, Edgar A Pask, joined the Royal Air Force and was seconded to the Institute of Aviation Medicine at Farnborough. His task was to investigate the causes of death in airmen who had baled out over the North Sea. As described in Chapter 5, he courageously volunteered to be deeply anaesthetized with ether and thrown into a swimming pool to test new designs of lifejacket. But he also became concerned with the effectiveness of the manual methods of artificial ventilation, and he and a colleague, John Roberts, were anaesthetized and intubated by Professor RR Macintosh and his First Assistant WW Mushin so that other methods of artificial ventilation could be tested. It was shown that blowing into the tracheal tube produced deeper breaths than any of the manual methods then in vogue.[7] But these investigators also realized that in the absence of a tracheal tube, the tongue would fall back and block the airway, and that this might impair the effectiveness of manual methods of artificial ventilation in the unconscious patient.

The importance of the airway

The breakthrough came in the 1950s, when James Elam and his anesthesiologist colleagues in Buffalo, New York, were asked to investigate methods of providing artificial ventilation to nerve gas casualties. They measured blood carbon dioxide and oxygen levels using the laborious van Slyke technique (which was also used by Astrup in the 1952 polio epidemic in Copenhagen), and showed that expired air resuscitation given via a face mask could provide adequate ventilation in unconscious subjects, providing that a clear airway could be maintained.[8,9] In 1958, Peter Safar, Archer Gordon, and other anesthesiologists in the USA, confirmed these findings and described in detail how the airway should be maintained.[10,11] A year later, Henning Ruben, a Danish anaesthetist, pointed out that in most patients the airway could be kept open by tilting the head backwards, while Safar and his colleagues published X-ray pictures showing how the anaesthetist's trick of tilting the head back and pushing the jaw forward could prevent the airway being obstructed by the tongue. Thereafter, this manoeuvre became an integral component of the resuscitation drill.[12]

As is customary with most medical advances, it took some time for mouth-to-mouth ventilation to be accepted. It is not pleasant to have to provide the kiss-of-life to an aged individual with bad breath and a beard, and there is always a risk of cross-infection, but it eventually became apparent that the advantages were so great that it had to be accepted as the method of choice. But it was only after much lobbying in the early 1960s that official bodies such as the Red Cross, the police and the ambulance services finally adopted mouth-to-mouth ventilation as the primary method of resuscitation in the UK.

One of the most important adjuncts to mouth-to-mouth ventilation is the self-inflating bag (Figure 16.2). This was developed by Henning Ruben,* when there was a transport strike that prevented oxygen supplies reaching Danish Hospitals in 1954. The bag is moulded so that

---

* Henning Ruben (1914–2004) financed his training as a dentist by working as a professional dancer. He practised as a dentist in Copenhagen from 1939 to 1943, but his partisan activities forced him to make a nocturnal crossing to neutral Sweden in a fishing boat. While in Sweden, he supported himself by working as a dentist, magician and thought-reader. He qualified in medicine in 1946, and subsequently trained as an anaesthetist in Sweden. Among his other inventions were a foot-operated suction pump and a resuscitation training manikin.[13]

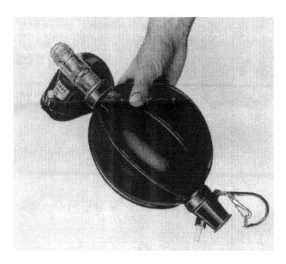

Figure 16.2 The self-inflating resuscitation bag invented by Henning Ruben. Oxygen can be added to the inlet of the bag, and the air/oxygen mixture is delivered to the patient through the Ruben non-rebreathing valve at the opposite end. (Reprinted from *Resuscitation* **64**, Baskett P, Images in resuscitation: Henning Ruben and the self inflating bag, 251–2, Copyright 2005, with permission from Elsevier.)

it rests in the inflated position and is thus always full of air. The air is sucked in through a non-return valve at one end, and when the bag is compressed, the air is driven into the lungs through the non-rebreathing valve at the other end. This valve switches to the expiratory position while the bag is refilling. Although oxygen can be added to the inspired gas, the value of the bag is that it provides a means of inflating the lungs when no supply of oxygen is available. It is thus of immense value in the emergency situation and has saved countless lives.[13]

Restarting the heart

To differentiate the sudden arrest of the heart from the normal pattern of death, we define a cardiac arrest as *a sudden and unexpected failure of the heart to provide an adequate cerebral circulation in a patient who is not suffering from a progressive and irrecoverable disease.*

Since treatment can only be effective if it is instituted quickly, diagnosis is based on the presence of just four clinical signs: unconsciousness, an absent pulse, respiratory arrest and dilated pupils that do not constrict when a light is shone in the eye. These signs provide a clear indication that the heart is not ejecting enough blood to keep the brain cells alive, and that resuscitation must be started immediately, but they do not tell us *why* the heart is not ejecting blood. In about 40% of cardiac arrests, the heart is in asystole, and in 60% of cases, it is in ventricular fibrillation. Since the treatment of these two conditions differs, it is necessary to determine which has caused the arrest as soon as an effective artificial respiration and circulation has been provided.

Internal cardiac compression

By the late 1950s, we were able to provide effective artificial ventilation either by mouth-to-mouth ventilation or by using an anaesthetic breathing system to deliver breaths of oxygen to a tube in the trachea, and we had the ability to defibrillate the heart if it was in ventricular fibrillation. However, fibrillation could only be diagnosed by connecting an electrocardiograph to the patient or by visualizing the heart. There were very few electrocardiographs at that time, so the standard treatment of cardiac arrest was to open the chest or abdomen and compress the heart manually. If the heart was seen to be in ventricular fibrillation, it was defibrillated, but if it was in asystole, drugs such as calcium and adrenaline (epinephrine) were injected into the heart to stimulate cardiac contraction.[14] Not surprisingly, such a heroic scenario was only enacted in the hospital, and then usually only in the operating theatre. Although I (KS) carried out a successful open-chest resuscitation in a corridor, the onlookers were not so accustomed to the sight of blood as today's television audiences, and the Matron politely requested that I should abandon my attempts at resuscitation in public places because the sight upset the visitors.

External cardiac compression

The real breakthrough came in 1960, when Kouvenhoven, Jude and Knickerbocker in the USA described how rhythmical pressure on the front of the chest could compress the heart between the breastbone and the spine.[15] They showed that this technique could force blood out of the heart into the aorta, and so into the coronary arteries and the rest of the circulation. It could thus provide a temporary supply of oxygen to the brain until the normal heartbeat could be restored. This technique was called external or closed-chest cardiac compression, and it revolutionized the treatment of cardiac arrest.

The development of mouth-to-mouth resuscitation and external cardiac compression was important for two reasons. First, resuscitation now became a simple procedure that could be started immediately, and in almost any environment, by anyone who witnessed the respiratory or cardiac arrest. Second, the institution of effective artificial ventilation and circulation of blood prevented further brain damage and so provided time for more definitive treatment to be effected. Even in hospital, it is not possible to site an expensive electrocardiograph and defibrillator close to every patient, so there is frequently a delay while the 'crash cart' is brought to the patient and definitive treatment is carried out. Outside hospital, the usual source of this equipment is the paramedic ambulance, and this too may take some minutes to arrive at the scene of the arrest. When the electrocardiograph is attached to the patient, the paramedic, doctor or nurse can determine whether the heart is in arrest or fibrillation. They can then carry out electrical defibrillation by passing a brief electric shock through large electrodes placed on the outside of the chest. In some cases, cardiac compression causes the heart to restart spontaneously, but if it does not, drugs can be administered either by an intravenous drip or by direct injection into the heart cavities through the chest wall.

The resuscitation team

In-hospital training

Because the technique of clearing and maintaining the airway is the first thing that anaesthetists learn, and because anaesthetists are skilled in inserting tubes into the trachea and in ventilating the lungs, it was natural that they should be among the first to teach the techniques of resuscitation to other doctors, nurses and paramedical staff. It is now standard practice for every hospital to have a rapid-response resuscitation team, usually with an anaesthetist as the coordinator, and to have electrocardiographs, defibrillators and cardiac drugs placed at strategic points around the hospital. Such a service results in a significant survival rate.[16]

Training of first-aid workers

The Norwegians have led the world in training schoolchildren and other members of the public in techniques of resuscitation. One of the most active protagonists was the industrialist Asmand Laerdal in Stavanger, and in the early 1960s he produced the inflatable doll called 'Resusci-Anne'. This doll has a moulded face and nasopharynx with an airway connected to model lungs, and the lungs can only be inflated if the rescuer maintains a clear airway by holding the head and chin in the correct position.

There are now many different manikins that can be used for training (Figure 16.3). Some have artificial hearts and arteries so that those performing cardiac compression can check that they are doing it effectively. Manikins such as Resusci-Anne are remarkably lifelike and have proven to be immensely valuable not only in initial training, but, even more importantly, in checking that operators have retained their skills and can still perform resuscitation effectively. The maintenance of high levels of competence is one of the major problems for those organizing the resuscitation services, and many anaesthetists accept this rather irksome, repetitive task as a very necessary part of their job.

Paramedic training

The successful treatment of cardiac arrest outside hospital has been mainly due to the provision of paramedic ambulances that are equipped with apparatus for intubation and ventilation of the lungs, electrocardiographs, defibrillators, and cardiac drugs. These ambulances are staffed by highly trained personnel who not only can carry out the primary resuscitation techniques, but can also insert intravenous infusions, pass tubes into the trachea so that the lungs can be ventilated

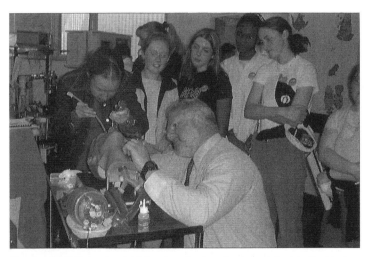

Figure 16.3 British schoolchildren learning how to pass a tube into the trachea on a training manikin. (Reproduced with the kind permission of the trainer, Dr Keith Stevens, the Wirral Health Authority Trust, Merseyside, and the Royal College of Anaesthetists.)

with oxygen, and then provide ongoing treatment of the cardiac condition. Peter Baskett, a Bristol anaesthetist, pioneered this type of training, and now most of these paramedic personnel receive intensive theoretical training from anaesthetists, cardiologists and doctors who work in accident and emergency departments, and they then gain practical experience with anaesthetists in the operating theatres.[17,18]

So where is the anaesthetist in the middle of all that mayhem on the television? He or she is the one who is quietly intubating the trachea, ventilating the lungs with oxygen, setting up an intravenous infusion, injecting drugs and monitoring the patient's condition. All the rest will be running the storyline.

References

1. Baker AB. The early days of expired air resuscitation. In: Atkinson RS, Boulton TB, eds, *The History of Anaesthesia*. London: Royal Society of Medicine, 1989: 372–4.
2. Tossack W. Man dead in appearance recovered by distending the lungs with air. In: *Medical Essays and Observations*. Edinburgh: J Fothergill, 1744. See also Fothergill J. Observations on a case report published in the last volume the Medical Essays etc of recovering a man dead in appearance by distending the lungs with air. *Philosophical Transactions of the Royal Society of London* 1756;**10**(abridged):968–71.
3. Brandt L, Gindi M El, Duda D, Ellmauer S. The development of organised emergency medicine in the18th century. In: Atkinson RS, Boulton TB, eds. *The History of Anaesthesia*. London: Royal Society of Medicine, 1989: 382–5.
4. Brandt L, Duda D, Gindi M El. The first instruments for resuscitation. In: Atkinson RS, Boulton TB, eds. *The History of Anaesthesia*. London: Royal Society of Medicine, 1989: 375–382.
5. Leroy J. Rechérches sur l'asphyxie. *Journal de Physiologie* 1827;**7**:45–65 and 1828;**8**:97–135.
6. Waters RM, Bennett JH. Artificial respiration: comparison of manual maneuvres. *Anesthesia and Analgesia* 1936;**15**:151–4.
7. Macintosh RR, Mushin WW. Pulmonary exchange during artificial respiration. *British Medical Journal* 1946;**1**:908–9.
8. Elam JO, Brown ES, Elder JD. Artificial ventilation by mouth-to-mask method. A study of the respiratory gas exchange of paralysed paralysed patients ventilated by operator's expired air. *New England Journal of Medicine* 1954;**250**:749–54.
9. Elam JO, Greene DG, Brown ES, Clements JA. Oxygen cost and carbon dioxide exchange and energy cost of expired air resuscitation. *Journal of the American Medical Association* 1958;**167**:328–34.
10. Safar P. Ventilatory efficiency of mouth-to-mouth artificial respiration. *Journal of the American Medical Association* 1958;**167**:335–41.
11. Safar P, Escarraga LA, Elam JO. A comparison of the mouth-to mouth and mouth-to airway methods of artificial respiration with the chest-pressure arm-lift methods. *New England Journal of Medicine* 1958;**258**:671–7.

12. Safar P, Escarraga LA, Chang F. Upper airway obstruction in the unconscious patient. *Journal of Applied Physiology* 1959;**14**:760–4.
13. Baskett P, Zorab J. Henning Ruben MD FFARCS(I), FFARCS. The Ruben valve and the AMBU bag. *Resuscitation* 2003;**56**:123–7.
14. Jude JR. Origins and development of cardiopulmonary resuscitation. In: Atkinson RS, Boulton TB, eds. *The History of Anaesthesia*. London: Royal Society of Medicine, 1989: 452–64.
15. Kouwenhoven WB, Jude JR, Knickerbocker GG. Closed chest cardiac massage. *Journal of the American Medical Association* 1960;**173**:1064–7.
16. Sykes MK, Orr DS. Cardio-pulmonary resuscitation. A report on two years' experience. *Anaesthesia* 1966;**21**:363–71.
17. Baskett PJ, Diamond AW, Cochrane DF. Urban mobile resuscitation: training and service. *British Journal of Anaesthesia* 1976;**48**:377–85.
18. Basket PJ. Uses of anaesthesia. The anaesthetist in the accident and emergency service. *British Medical Journal* 1980;**281**:287–9.

17 The search for a better inhalation agent

John Bunker, when Chairman of the Department of Anesthesia at Stanford University, received a phone call one morning in 1962 from the Director of Pathology at the Sutter Community Hospital in Sacramento, California. Could a new anaesthetic, halothane, damage the liver, he asked? A 16-year-old girl had died in liver failure 13 days following halothane anaesthesia for surgical repair of a lacerated wrist she had suffered in falling through a glass window. At postmortem, 80% of the liver was destroyed. The fatal outcome was strikingly similar to liver death after anaesthesia with chloroform. The phone call from Sacramento, and reports of a small number of similar deaths, catalysed a national study of the toxic effects of anaesthetic agents.[1]

Following the discovery of the anaesthetic effects of diethyl ether in 1846, medical practitioners began to seek better inhalation anaesthetic agents – a search that continues today. Within a year, James Simpson, the Professor of Midwifery at the University of Edinburgh, dissatisfied with the side-effects of ether in childbirth, began to look for an alternative. Simpson was at first interested in the possible anaesthetic properties of ethylene dibromide. He had intended to inhale the vapour himself, but did not proceed when he discovered that two rabbits used to assess the safety of the agent had died.[2] Simpson, together with colleagues, then indulged in self-experimentation with a number of other volatile drugs, one of which was chloroform, as recounted in Chapter 1. Championed by Simpson, chloroform largely supplanted ether in the UK, but its popularity declined after the 1870s when it was recognized that chloroform could cause sudden cardiac death and liver failure.

Seventy years were to pass before the anaesthetic effects of ethylene gas were seriously explored, initially in mice, rabbits and dogs, and then in man. Its potential as an anaesthetic was recognized by chance, as occurs so often with medical discoveries. The anaesthetic effect of ethylene was traced to a report of its dramatic impact in the floral industry. '*During the early part of 1908 severe losses were sustained by carnation growers shipping their products into Chicago, because of the fact that these flowers, when placed in the greenhouses, would "go to sleep", whereas the buds already showing petals failed to open*'.[3] The closing of flowering carnations had been traced to a leak of illuminating gas in a greenhouse, and was ultimately found to be the result of contamination of the gas by ethylene. If ethylene induced sleep in a flowering plant, perhaps it would do the same in humans. Ethylene was a little more potent than nitrous oxide and could produce unconsciousness when given with normal concentrations of oxygen. It briefly supplanted nitrous oxide in America, but it is highly explosive when mixed with air or oxygen, and by 1933 over 20 explosions had been reported, so few persisted with its use.

While the use of ethylene was decreasing, another potentially explosive inhalation anaesthetic, cyclopropane, was introduced. Its anaesthetic properties had been demonstrated in animals by George WH Lucas and VE Henderson of Toronto University in 1929,[4] and Professor Henderson himself volunteered to be the first subject to be anaesthetized with the gas. Cyclopropane was a relatively non-irritant and highly potent gas that could be given with high concentrations of oxygen. Induction and recovery were rapid, and it did not lower blood pressure, so it was frequently used for patients in shock. It was also popular in thoracic surgery because it depressed the respiratory centre, enabling the anaesthetist to control ventilation and thus to afford the surgeon a quiet operating field. But, like ethylene, it is highly explosive when mixed with air or oxygen, and is no longer manufactured as an anaesthetic.

Another drug that was used predominantly in the UK from the 1940s until the 1960s was trichloroethylene (Trilene). This had been used in industry as a degreasing and dry-cleaning agent since its discovery at the end of the 19th century. It was observed that, when inhaled, it relieved the pain of trigeminal neuralgia ('*tic douloureux*'), and this led to its use in anaesthesia. It is non-explosive and, although not potent enough to be used as an anaesthetic by itself, was used in combination with nitrous oxide for minor surgical procedures. It was also used to provide pain relief during labour.

Recognition of the need for a safer anaesthetic agent initiated a wide search for an anaesthetic of intermediate potency: a drug more potent than nitrous oxide to allow it to be administered with an adequate concentration of oxygen; a drug less potent than chloroform, cyclopropane or ether, to lessen the risk of overdosage and cardiac depression. In addition, it should be chemically inert and non-flammable. The search for such an anaesthetic was aided by the already considerable body of experience and theory on the relationship of chemical structure to function. As it turned out, the necessary constraints imposed severe limitations on the choice of chemical compounds. To achieve a compound with physical properties that were appropriate for a general anaesthetic, it was necessary to choose one based on a hydrocarbon. To render the hydrocarbon non-explosive, it was necessary to substitute halogen atoms for hydrogen atoms. The long search led to a number of new drugs with anaesthetic properties, the most promising being halothane, 2-bromo-2-chloro-1,1,1-trifluroroethane. Halothane, distributed under the trade name 'Fluothane', was synthesized at Imperial Chemical Industries in Manchester, but it soon became apparent that it was not a drug of 'intermediate potency', but was more potent than ether and almost as potent as chloroform.[5]

Halothane had several marked clinical advantages,[6] the most notable of which was a more rapid induction than that experienced with other inhalation anaesthetics, and, combined with curare, it appeared to be nearly the ideal anaesthetic.[7] Its clinical performance was so clearly superior to anaesthetics then in general use that it quite literally swept the country – the UK, that is – followed within two years by every other country in the Western world. By 1962, it had been administered to several million patients undergoing surgery, and was considered the 'anaesthetic of choice'.

Halothane was introduced to clinical anaesthesia in the UK in 1956 and in the USA in 1958. Careful consideration had been given to the possibility that halothane, in common with other hydrocarbons incorporating halogens (chlorine, bromine or fluorine), might damage the liver. Carbon tetrachloride, once used in dry cleaning, is well known as a potential cause of fatal liver injury, the anaesthetic chloroform only slightly less so. But in its early years of use, halothane demonstrated no evidence of liver injury and appeared to have an impressive record of safety.

But there were, in addition to the 16-year-old patient described at the beginning of the chapter,[1] a small number of other reports of patients who had suffered fatal liver failure following halothane anaesthesia. The question that needed to be addressed was whether the handful of similar deaths that had come to light represented just the tip of the iceberg, or were simply an extremely rare and sporadic complication, statistically of no significance. Was this, in other words, a public health problem of major proportions – one that needed to be assessed in the broader context of surgical and anaesthetic risks as a whole?

There was widespread concern among surgeons and physicians, as well as among anaesthetists. Less than a year had passed since the thalidomide tragedy. Americans had largely escaped the tragedy of phocomelia, the congenital loss of arms or legs, since thalidomide had not been approved by the Food and Drug Administration (FDA) in Washington. And there was concern that FDA approval of halothane might be revoked, while the evidence for or against the safety of halothane was fragmentary at best.

Suddenly, there were reports of a dozen cases of fatal liver failure after halothane anaesthesia, and another witch-hunt was on. This time, the anesthesiologists were ready. Halothane had proven itself clinically in several million administrations, but the possibility of serious toxicity had been raised. It was clearly of public health concern, sufficiently serious to justify a major clinical investigation. Convinced of the urgent need to assess the safety of halothane, the National Academy of Sciences/National Research Council in Washington and its Committee on Anesthesia were able to obtain funding from the National Institutes of Health in Bethesda, Maryland, for the large-scale study that would be necessary.

It was recognized that the necessary data could probably be obtained only in a very large series of carefully matched surgical patients, with the patients being randomly allocated to receive anaesthesia with halothane or with other drugs. To plan, organize, and conduct such a study, the National Academy was able to enlist the assistance of a distinguished panel of physicians and statisticians to form what became the Subcommittee on the National Halothane Study.

The primary objective of the Study was to compare halothane with other general anaesthetics regarding the incidence of fatal massive hepatic necrosis. An equally important objective was to compare mortality from all causes – surgical as well as anaesthetic – because it was recognized that, even if halothane were found to be responsible for death from hepatic necrosis more often than with other anaesthetics, the incidence would probably be very small compared with overall operative mortality. Indeed, a slight superiority in overall survival of patients who had received halothane could well outweigh any excess of deaths resulting from hepatic necrosis. This was, in fact, one of the most important findings of the study.

The randomized trial was never completed. In the first month of randomization, there was a new case of fatal liver necrosis, and the trial was cancelled on ethical grounds. How could one justify the 'experimental' administration of halothane to patients in view of its imputed risk? Ironically, the widespread clinical use of halothane continued while the Halothane Committee searched for other ways to answer the question of whether the use of halothane was linked to fatal liver failure. With the prospective clinical trial precluded, a retrospective study of past data was reluctantly accepted as the only alternative.

It was asked at the outset why the Committee had not simply recommended stopping the use of halothane, as many surgeons and other physicians had urged. The answer was that the numerators were known, but not the denominator. The numerators consisted of randomly reported instances of fatal liver injury following the administration of halothane, and thus were incomplete. The total number of patients who had received halothane, the denominator, was unknown. What the research committee could conclude thus far was that there had been some unfortunate but rare deaths. '*Before indicting a procedure*,' a member of the committee wrote, '*we should compare its performance with those of competitive procedures used in similar circumstances. With numerator only data we have only the cases with bad outcomes and thus no rate to compare with other rates for other procedures*'.[8]

The study as it was finally carried out was a remarkable feat of what was, at that time, a miracle of modern computer science and data processing. Sections from the livers of just under 1000 patients in whom liver injury might have contributed to death were examined. The hospital records of 17 000 patients and autopsy reports of 17 000 were reviewed, all collected from a total of 865 000 patients undergoing anaesthesia and surgery in the 34 hospitals that participated in the study.[9]

When the study had been completed, 82 cases of massive hepatic necrosis had been identified, the majority occurring in patients undergoing high-risk surgery. The incidence of massive hepatic necrosis after administration of halothane was virtually the same as that after administration of thiopental and nitrous oxide, more than that after ether anaesthesia, and considerably less than that following the administration of cyclopropane. There were only three patients in whom there was fatal liver necrosis following 367 000 operations that were defined as 'low-risk'.

Since completion of the study, it has been established that halothane can, rarely, cause liver damage. The possibility of a genetic predisposition was raised when three pairs of closely related women of similar ethnic origin were found to have suffered hepatitis following halothane anaesthesia.[10] Further evidence came from two anaesthetists who suffered relapsing hepatitis. They had recovered when removed from the operating theatre exposure to anesthetic vapours, but had suffered an acute relapse when subjected to a brief diagnostic 'challenge' to halothane. A number of reasonably comparable patients who suffered liver injury following repeated exposures to halothane lent further support to a syndrome that has come to be known as 'halothane hepatitis'.

By the time that the National Halothane Study had been completed, however, there had been too few instances of fatal liver injury to establish 'halothane hepatitis' as a clinical syndrome. What could be stated with confidence was that the danger of halothane-induced liver injury did not constitute a serious public health problem. Indeed, the overall death rate following surgery conducted under halothane was less on average than that of surgery under other anaesthetic agents. It was concluded that halothane anaesthesia, rather than being dangerous, had a remarkable record of safety.

Recognition of the rarity of halothane-induced liver injury has prompted a re-examination of the historical evidence for 'delayed chloroform toxicity'.[11] In 1912, the Committee on Anesthesia of the American Medical Association advised that the use of chloroform as an anaesthetic could no longer be justified. The advice was based on the conclusion that delayed chloroform poisoning 'follows in a by no means inconsiderable percentage of cases'. But there were no data from which to estimate its incidence. There had been isolated case reports of liver injury or death following chloroform, even as there were in the years leading up to the National Halothane Study. Without the Halothane Study, halothane might have suffered the same fate.

Concern that liver damage might follow the administration of halothane eventually caused most anaesthetists to switch to enflurare and, later, isoflurane, two other potent and non-explosive agents that were also relatively insoluble in blood and therefore had relatively short induction and recovery times (Figure 17.1). The introduction of such agents facilitated another major advance in medical care: day-case surgery. Although this concept had originated in Glasgow at the beginning of the 20th century, it was the introduction of short-acting anaesthetic agents that provided the impetus for its rapid development over the last 30 years (see Chapter 19).

Afterword

The National Halothane Study was designed to study a particular, and, as it turned out, rare anaesthetic complication; a secondary objective was to compare surgical mortality when conducted under differing anaesthetic agents. In the process of pursuing these twin objectives, a comprehensive catalogue of surgical deaths was generated. This provided new information on risks and outcomes following surgery, and more

Advances in anaesthesia

Curare
Pethidine

Lignocaine
Recovery wards
Induced hypotension

Poisoning units
Pain clinics

Manual IPPV
Mechanical ventilators
Two-part Diploma in Anaesthetics
Obstetric analgesia with trichloroethylene
Patient transport
Halothane

Intensive care units

In-hospital cardiac arrest service
Entonox for obstetric analgesia

Bupivacaine

Community resuscitation training

Enflurane

Isoflurane

Propofol (1977) LMA (1988)

Other advances

Penicillin

Streptomycin
Closed-heart surgery
National Health Service
Faculty of Anaesthetists

WHO anaesthesia course
Copenhagen polio epidemic
Confidential Enquiry into Maternal Deaths

Respiratory care units
Induced hypothermia for cardiac surgery

Polio vaccine

Open-heart surgery (UK)

Blood gas analysis
Closed chest cardiac compression
Coronary care units
Kidney transplantation
Liver transplantation

Gate theory of pain

Heart transplantation

Timeline: 1945, 1950, 1955, 1960, 1965, 1970

Figure 17.1 Time chart (1945–70) showing the relationship between the introduction of new inhalation anaesthetics (in bold) and other advances in anaesthesia and related areas of medicine. Two other new short-acting inhalation agents, desflurane and sevoflurane, were introduced in the 1980s and have been widely used for day-case surgery. IPPV, intermittent positive-pressure ventilation; LMA, laryngeal mask airway (which has largely replaced the tracheal tube for routine anaesthesia).

particularly the opportunity to compare hospitals for their surgical successes and failures. It was the National Halothane Study, in fact, that initiated the intense scrutiny of medical and surgical practice, reports of which we now see in the daily press.

References

1. Bunker JP, Blumenfeld CM. Liver necrosis after halothane anesthesia. *New England Journal of Medicine* 1963;**268**:531–4.
2. Youngson AJ. *The Scientific Revolution in Victorian Medicine*, London: Croom Helm, 1979.
3. Luckhardt AB, Carter JB. The physiological effects of ethylene. *Journal of the American Medical Association* 1923;**80**:765–70.
4. Lucas GHW, Henderson VE. New anaesthetic gas: cyclopropane; preliminary report. *Canadian Medical Association Journal* 1929;**21**:173–5.
5. Suckling CW. Some chemical and physical factors in the development of Fluothane. *British Journal of Anaesthesia* 1957;**29**:466–72.
6. Raventos J. Action of Fluothane – a new volatile anaesthetic. *British Journal of Pharmacology* 1956;**11**:394–410.
7. Johnstone M. Human cardiovascular response to Fluothane anaesthesia. *British Journal of Anaesthesia* 1956;**28**:392–410.
8. Mosteller F. Unpublished manuscript.
9. Bunker JP, Forrest WH, Mosteller F, Vandam LD, eds. *The National Halothane Study*. Bethesda, MD: National Institutes of Health, 1969.
10. Hoft RH, Bunker JP, Goodman HI, Gregory PB. Halothane hepatitis in three pairs of closely related women. *New England Journal of Medicine* 1981;**304**:1023–4.
11. Dykes MHM. The early years: 1846–1912. In: *Anesthesia and the Liver. International Anesthesiology Clinics* 1970;**8**(2):175–87.

18 The pursuit of safety

What are the risks of having an anaesthetic? Anaesthetists make mistakes, as do others, but can we prevent accidents and, if so, how? On the 22 April 1982, the American television series '20/20' aired a program entitled 'The Deep Sleep: 6,000 Will Die or Suffer Brain Damage'. The announcer's opening words were that *'if you are going to go into anesthesia, you are going on a long trip and you should not do it, if you can avoid it in any way. General anesthesia is safe most of the time, but there are dangers from human error, carelessness and a crucial shortage of anesthesiologists'.*[1] With approximately 20 million anaesthetics and operations performed in the USA annually, the estimate would reflect a rate of death or brain damage of approximately one in 3300. How accurate was the television estimate? Assuming that the order of magnitude is roughly correct, what remedial action has been taken, and has there been improvement in the intervening two decades?

Determining the incidence of mortality directly attributable to anaesthesia has been an elusive goal, and estimates vary widely. The Washington-based Institute of Medicine, in its seminal book *To Err is Human*, published in 2000, states that over the past 20 years, anaesthesia mortality rates have been reduced from 2 deaths per 10 000 to 1 death per 100 000 anaesthetics.[2] The Joint Commission on the Accreditation of Hospitals in America cites the same figures. The rates are, at best, speculative. A more recent review of published data reports that an *'anesthesia-related mortality rate, as determined by peer review, has been stable over the past decade at approximately one death per 13,000 anesthetics'*.[3] What can be said is that an anaesthetic death is rare. If the correct rate were to be one in 13 000 today, this would mean that of 13 000 patients undergoing general anaesthesia for surgery, 12 999 would survive the administration of the anaesthetic.

These sound like very good odds. But why should there be any anaesthetic deaths at all? Surgical risk can be justified within the context of potential benefits, an increase in the length of life or an improvement in its quality, but surgical anaesthesia cannot be justified on these grounds. Anaesthetic deaths are unacceptable, and anaesthetists, from the first administrations in the mid-19th century, have been preoccupied with efforts to prevent them.

Anaesthetic deaths are rare, but when they do occur, is it the drug that is responsible or the way in which it is administered? The drugs now in use are safer than those available in the 19th and early 20th centuries. Nevertheless, as with therapeutic drugs prescribed elsewhere in the practice of medicine, there will always be some risk due to their inherent toxicity. Of greater concern today, however, is technical and human error.

The Critical Incident Study

Anaesthetic deaths have been subjected to intense scrutiny at traditional departmental conferences that review mortality. But in a busy hospital performing 10 000–20 000 operations a year, there might be only one or two such deaths a year, which is hardly an adequate basis on which to judge the nature of anaesthetic deaths in general, to explain them, and to formulate remedial policy. However, while there are very few deaths, there may be many 'near-misses', just as there are in aviation. The study of near-misses has been formalized as a research methodology, the analysis of 'critical incidents'. A critical incident is defined as 'an abnormal occurrence that, if not corrected, would probably have resulted in an adverse outcome or death'. Widely employed in the aircraft industry, it is equally apposite for the study of risk in anaesthesia. Its introduction for the study of anaesthesia risk by Jeffrey Cooper represented a milestone in the search for patient safety.

Cooper is an engineer in the Department of Anesthesia at the Massachusetts General Hospital in Boston. He was recruited in the early 1970s to join the department's Bioengineering Unit; together with other members of the unit, he was to be responsible for *'developing new instrumentation, particularly devices to support research, but also that might have direct clinical applications'* .[4] Their challenge was to design an anaesthesia delivery system that would prevent, or at least minimize, the occurrence of human error. Together with his colleagues, Cooper built a microprocessor-based system designed to eliminate human factor problems associated with anaesthesia delivery machines that had been fundamentally unchanged for the previous 50–75 years.[5]

The construction of their experimental electronic anaesthesia system was based on the assumption that technical flaws in the design of anaesthetic apparatus were largely responsible for errors in the provision of anaesthesia and that it should be possible to design equipment that would minimize, if not prevent, anaesthetic mishaps. To test this hypothesis, Cooper led a team of investigators to conduct a 'retrospective examination of the characteristics of human error and equipment failure in anaesthetic practice'. For this purpose, they conducted in-depth interviews of staff anaesthetists and residents in training, requesting them to report near-misses or critical incidents.

By mid-1970, after the first 25 pilot interviews, '*it became clear that equipment problems were not the major concern. Much more interesting were the myriad ways in which physicians and nurses could err in the administration of drugs, in diagnosis and in the exercise of judgement – all of which were intimately tied to the larger system in which they worked*'. In their first paper published in 1978, Cooper and his colleagues reported inadvertent breathing system disconnection, errors in gas flow settings and mistaken drug dosage as being the most frequent causes of a critical incident.[6]

The critical incident studies were initially carried out in a single hospital. They were subsequently expanded to include an additional three affiliated hospitals at Harvard University. Their findings, published in 1984,[7] led to the formulation of a set of recommendations for measures designed to prevent and detect major errors and equipment failures in anaesthesia management. These included additional technical training, improved supervision, improved organization, improvements in equipment design and the use of additional monitoring instrumentation.

Following the study of critical incidents, the Harvard anaesthesia departments devised specific, detailed, mandatory standards for use during anaesthesia at the nine component teaching hospitals.[8,9] The Harvard standards were widely debated at the time but are now accepted throughout the USA, and similar guidelines have been promulgated by the Association of Anaesthetists of Great Britain and Ireland, and by most of the organizations concerned with anaesthesia in other countries.

The adoption of the Harvard standards in its nine hospitals was followed by a dramatic improvement in malpractice liability experience. Writing in 1989, the lawyer James Holzer, Vice-President of the Risk Management Foundation in Cambridge, Massachusetts, could write that Harvard '*anesthesiologists will see their 1989 premiums cut by almost one-third over the previous year's rate*'.[10]

The Closed Claims Study

Malpractice liability insurance had become virtually unavailable for American anaesthetists in the 1970s, and this was followed by a crisis of affordability in the 1980s.The adoption of standards, together with other initiatives to improve the quality of anaesthetic care, resulted in an equally dramatic fall in malpractice claims. In 1984, the American Society of Anesthesiologists (ASA), concerned by rapidly escalating professional liability insurance premiums, had sought access to the closed claims files of several of the major insurers against medical malpractice. Between 1975 and 1978, anaesthesia injuries accounted for 3% of all paid claims but 11% of all dollars paid out.[10] Death accounted for 30% of injuries, brain damage 12% and nerve damage 18% in 1980.[11]

It was hoped that by determining the nature of injury for which compensation had been paid, remedial action could be designed and put into effect. The claims files of the insurance industry are normally guarded as 'business secrets', but in response to the crisis in malpractice claims, the National Association of Insurance Commissioners started to collect details of closed medical malpractice claims that were offered for professional medical review. When access to closed claims relating to anaesthesia was made available, the Closed Claims Study was initiated.

The Closed Claims Study was described by its proponents as '*a structural evaluation of anesthetic mishaps … to identify causes of anesthesia related injury and the contribution of substandard care to those injuries*'.[12] The study had many limitations, the most prominent of which was the absence of denominator data: injuries spoke for themselves and formed the numerator, but there was no way to determine the number of anaesthetics administered to serve as a denominator, from which the incidence of the injury could be estimated. But what the study was able to provide was a remarkable opportunity to analyse a large collection of anaesthetic mishaps, '*otherwise attainable only by laborious, expensive, time-consuming surveys*'.[13]

Traced over the two decades from the 1970s to 1990s, there was a very large decrease in claims. The proportion of claims for permanent disabling injuries fell from 65% of all claims to 42%, claims for death fell from 41% to 22%, and claims for brain damage from 15% to 10%.[11] And even by the time when the Closed Claims Study was being initiated, the US General Accounting Office reported that allegations of anaesthesia error had fallen to 5.6% of indemnity payments. By 1986–87, total claims for anaesthesia-related injury reported by one of the major insurance agencies had fallen to 3.5% of total claims.[10]

The Confidential Enquiries

In 1977, D Bruce Scott, an Edinburgh Consultant Anaesthetist who had been closely concerned with regional and obstetric anaesthesia for many years, wrote an editorial in the *British Journal of Anaesthesia* in which he recommended that a study similar to the Confidential Enquiry into Maternal Deaths (discussed in Chapter 21), should be set up to look at the problem of deaths during anaesthesia and surgery.[14] The suggestion was taken up by the Association of Anaesthetists, whose Council appointed a working party, chaired by Professor WW Mushin from Cardiff, to advise on the organization of the study. The Nuffield Provincial Hospitals Trust agreed to provide generous funding for three years and, for practical purposes, it was agreed to include about one-third of all the National Health Service (NHS) hospitals in the study. These were situated in Wales, Scotland and three English NHS Regions.

The central assessors appointed assessors in each region, and these appointed local correspondents in each hospital in collaboration with the local departments of anaesthesia. The correspondents identified patients who had died within six days of surgery, and sent separate letters and questionnaires to the surgeon and anaesthetist concerned, asking them to return these to the regional assessor.

The report, which was published in 1982, was based on 6060 deaths that were associated with 1 147 362 operations. JN Lunn (a Cardiff anaesthetist and Chairman of the Regional Assessor's Committee) and Professor Mushin concluded that:

'The overwhelming message of this report is that the process of anaesthesia is remarkably safe. Although one in 166 (0.6%) of patients die within 6 days of operation, only one in 10,000 dies totally as a result of anaesthesia. Thus the number of deaths totally attributable to anaesthesia is in the region of 280 per year in the United Kingdom ... the majority of these are probably preventable ... The events which have caused the deaths have not changed over 30 years'.[15]

Lunn and Mushin went on to list a number of deficiencies in the anaesthetic services in the NHS. Trainees were often left without adequate Consultant support; there was inadequate monitoring apparatus, insufficient consultation between surgeons and anaesthetists, inadequate preoperative preparation of the patient, and disregard by the surgeons of the implications of intercurrent disease in the patient; and, in 17.5% of the cases, the hospital had no recovery room.

The report received much media coverage and created quite a stir among anaesthetists and surgeons. The study stimulated interest in audit among the surgical community, and led to the setting up of a joint study supported by the Association of Anaesthetists and the Association of Surgeons of Great Britain and Ireland. This Confidential Enquiry into Perioperative Deaths (CEPOD) reported in 1987.[16] As a result of the widespread interest in this report, the government agreed to finance a National Confidential Enquiry into Perioperative Deaths (NCEPOD). This independent body was supported by both of the Associations and by both of the Royal Colleges and their Faculties. It issued regular reports that dealt with specific areas of surgical activity and concentrated attention on topical problems that needed to be addressed. These included the broader problems of provision of appropriate facilities, training and organization of the service, as well as those pertaining to the clinical problems of the specific area being studied.[17] The responsibility for this organization has now been transferred to the National Institute for Clinical Excellence (NICE) and the remit has been extended to include medical patients and primary care. The new body is still known as NCEPOD, but this acronym now stands for the National Confidential Enquiry into Patient Outcomes and Deaths.

An independent review of the Enquiry carried out in 1998 found that 1700 of 2195 Consultants stated that NCEPOD had changed their clinical practice in at least one way. Furthermore, managers are now provided with firm evidence justifying changes in clinical practice. For example, many hospitals have now provided an operating theatre dedicated to emergency care in order that patients and staff are not required to wait until the evening before the operation can be performed. This has reduced out-of-hours surgery and improved the supervision of junior staff.[18]

All of these studies led to the same conclusion: namely that the majority of deaths and complications were preventable. By this time, training had been greatly improved so the question was what else could be done to make anaesthesia safer?

The introduction of patient and equipment monitoring devices

Until the mid-1970s, most of the equipment used to make measurements in medicine was research-based and inadequate for clinical use. It did not include audible or visual alarms, for example, which are considered essential today. By the early 1980s, manufacturers were introducing microprocessors into medical equipment, and sophisticated apparatus for monitoring the patient's condition and anaesthetic machine function was beginning to appear in the marketplace (Figure 18.1). Analysis of

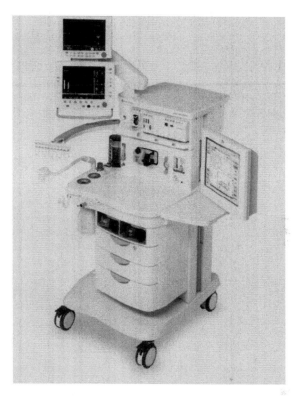

Figure 18.1 A modern anaesthetic machine: the Aisys (Anaesthesia Integrated System). This incorporates a mechanical ventilator, apparatus for measuring the gas pressures and the flow and composition of inspired and expired gases, and various alarm systems. The measured machine variables are displayed on one screen and the output from the monitors attached to the patient are displayed on a second screen. (Reproduced with permission from GE Healthcare, Hatfield, Hertfordshire, UK.)

insurance claims and critical incident data revealed that most incidents could have been avoided if adequate monitoring apparatus had been used. For example, data from the ASA Closed Claims Study showed that out of 624 claims of all types (excluding tooth injury), 193 were due to respiratory mishaps, of which 80 were classified as inadequate ventilation and 41 as inadvertent oesophageal intubation. The report concluded that 69% of the respiratory-related claims were judged to be preventable with better monitoring.

While there are a few die-hards who preach that clinical observation is more effective than the most expensive electronic device, there is no doubt that the provision and use of monitoring apparatus has had an enormous impact on patient safety, both in the operating room and in recovery, high-dependency and intensive care units. The early devices were plagued by many false alarms, but sophisticated software has now overcome many of these problems, and few anaesthetics are given without active monitors of anaesthetic machine and ventilator function, together with devices that monitor ventilation, oxygenation, circulation and other aspects of the patient's condition (Figure 18.2).

'Anesthesiologists have led the field' (Leape, 1994)[19]

Anaesthesia has been judged to be the leading medical speciality in terms of addressing issues of patient safety. This judgement comes from the Institute of Medicine in Washington, DC[2] and from the American surgeon Lucian Leape, a leader of the national, now international, movement to

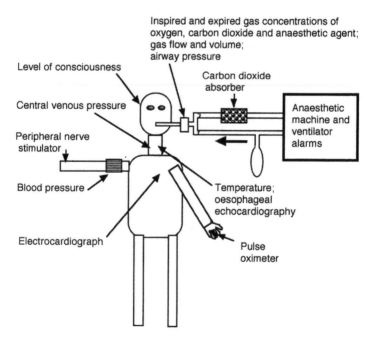

Figure 18.2 Routine monitoring employed during anaesthesia today.

address the issue of errors in medicine. Addressing the problem of errors in medicine, Leape wrote that *'unlike aviation, safety in medicine has never been institutionalized'*. Citing anaesthesia as an exception, he wrote that *'Anesthesiologists have led the field in recognizing system failures as causes of errors, in designing fail-safe systems, and in training to avoid errors'*.[19]

Why did the problem of medical errors and patient safety emerge in the USA, and why did anaesthesia in particular lead the way? Anaesthesia was among the medical specialities that had been most heavily hit by rising insurance premiums, more so in the USA but increasingly in the UK as well. The malpractice crisis galvanized the profession at all levels, including grassroots clinicians, to address seriously issues of patient safety. But why anaesthesia in particular? In a seminal article in the *British Medical Journal* entitled 'Anaesthesiology as a model for patient safety', the California anaesthetist David Gaba explained that:

'As anaesthesia care became more complex and technological and expanded to include intensive care it attracted a higher calibre of staff. Clinicians working in anaesthesiology tend to be risk averse' [primarily] *because anaesthesia can be dangerous and has no therapeutic benefit of its own. Anaesthesiology also attracted individuals with backgrounds in engineering* [who] *found models for safety in anaesthesia in other hazardous technological pursuits, including aviation'*.[20]

In collaboration with Jeffrey Cooper, whose groundbreaking studies of 'critical incidents' we discussed above, Gaba wrote that anaesthesia had widely adopted guidelines in monitoring, carried out in-depth analyses of malpractice claims, addressed the widespread problem of fatigue, developed simulators for real-time training and tackled problems of human error.

Anaesthesia, administered to facilitate surgery, does not, by definition, save lives. But surgical anaesthesia does save countless lives, indirectly, by allowing surgeons to perform operations not feasible in an earlier era – operations that do save lives.

References

1. Tomlin J. The Deep Sleep. 6,000 Will Die or Suffer Brain Damage. Chicago: WLS TV '20/20', 22 April, 1982 – quoted by Pierce E. The 34th Rovenstine Lecture: 40 Years Behind the Mask: Safety Revisited. *Anesthesiology* 1996;**84**:965–75.
2. Kohn LT, Corrigan JM, Donaldson MS, eds. *To Err is Human: Building a Safer Health System*. Washington, DC, National Academy Press, 2000.

3. Lagasse RS. Anesthesia safety: model or myth? *Anesthesiology* 2002;**97**:1609–17.
4. Cooper JB. An accidental life: patient safety and biomedical engineering. In: Kitz RJ, ed. *'This is No Humbug!' Reminiscences of the Department of Anesthesia at the Massachusetts General Hospital – A History*. Boston: privately published, 2003.
5. Cooper JB, Newbower RS. Moore JW, et al. A new anesthesia delivery system. *Anesthesiology* 1978;**49**:310–18.
6. Cooper JB, Newbower RS, Long CD, McPeek B. Preventable anesthesia mishaps: a study of human factors. *Anesthesiology* 1978;**49**:399–406.
7. Cooper JB, Newbower RS, Kitz RJ. An analysis of major errors and equipment eailures in anesthesia management: considerations for prevention and detection. *Anesthesiology* 1984;**60**:34–42.
8. Eichhorn JH, Cooper JB, Cullen DJ et al. Standards for patient monitoring during anesthesia at Harvard Medical School. *Journal of the American Medical Association* 1986;**256**:1017–20.
9. Eichhorn JH. Prevention of intraoperative anesthesia accidents and related severe injury through safety monitoring. *Anesthesiology* 1989;**70**:572–7.
10. Holzer JF. Liability insurance issues in anesthesiology. *International Anesthesiology Clinics* 1989;**27**:205–12.
11. Lee LA, Domino KB. The Closed Claims Project: Has it influenced anesthetic practice and outcome? *Anesthesiology Clinics of North America* 2002;**20**:485–501.
12. Cheney FW. The American Society of Anesthesiologists Closed Claim Project: What have we learned, how has it affected practice, and how will it affect practice in the future? *Anesthesiology* 1999;**91**:552–6.
13. Keats AS. The Closed Claims Study. *Anesthesiology* 1990;**73**:199–201.
14. Scott DB. Editorial. Deaths associated with anaesthesia. *British Journal of Anaesthesia* 1977;**49**:95–6.
15. Lunn JN, Mushin WW. *Mortality Associated with Anaesthesia*. London: The Nuffield Provincial Hospitals Trust, 1982.
16. Lunn JN, Devlin HB. Lessons from the National Confidential Enquiry into Perioperative Deaths in three NHS regions. *Lancet* 1987;**ii**:1384–6.
17. Lunn JN. The history and achievements of the National Confidential Enquiry into Perioperative Deaths. *Journal of Quality in Clinical Practice* 1998;**18**:29–35.
18. Mayor S. Changing practice. *British Medical Journal* 2004;**328**:248.
19. Leape LL. Errors in medicine. *Journal of the American Medical Association* 1994;**272**:1851–7.
20. Gaba DM. Anaesthesiology as a model for patient safety in health care. *British Medical Journal* 2000;**320**:785–8.

19 The fast track: sedation and day-case surgery

It costs a lot of money to keep a patient in hospital, and patients dislike the experience. For many, the answer is to take the fast track and to undergo surgery as a day case.

'Fast-tracking' is now the buzz word in medical care: the shorter the time the patient spends in hospital, the less will be the cost, and the smaller the chance of picking up an opportunistic infection. The theory is simple, but the implementation more difficult. Anaesthetists have responded to the challenge by two developments: the use of sedation to facilitate a wide variety of medical and radiological investigations, and the creation of day-case (ambulatory) surgical units. These innovations owe much of their success to the new drugs and techniques of anaesthesia that have been introduced over the past 30 years, and so bring our story into the 21st century.

Sedation

Sedation reduces anxiety and discomfort. The patient may sleep, but should be rousable. Some sedative drugs also produce amnesia, so that the patient has little memory of any procedures that take place during the period of sedation. Sedative drugs were first used as a premedication to prepare the patient for operation, but, in recent years, sedation has largely replaced general anaesthesia for many medical and radiological investigations, and for other procedures that may produce discomfort but not severe pain.

Premedication

The use of sedative drugs to calm patients before operation started at the beginning of the 20th century and soon became routine. The drugs most commonly employed were various injectable preparations of opium, and these were usually given with an injection of atropine or hyoscine (scopolamine). The opiate produced sedation, augmented the analgesia provided by nitrous oxide, and also helped to relieve pain after operation. The atropine was used to decrease oral secretions so that they were not aspirated into the lungs, but, as atropine had no sedative action, hyoscine was used more frequently. This drug not only decreased secretions but also had sedative, antiemetic and amnesic actions. Barbiturate drugs were given when the anaesthetist wished to avoid an injection.

Because of the high incidence of barbiturate poisoning, other oral preparations were introduced. In the 1960s, a combination of an opiate with an antihistamine drug such as promethazine (Phenergan) became popular, but this often produced prolonged somnolence after operation. During the last 30–40 years, benzodiazepine drugs such as diazepam, midazolam, lorazepam and temazepam have been used increasingly, because they produce effective sedation and amnesia, and have few other side-effects.

Sedation techniques for investigations and surgery

During the past half-century, many new medical and radiological investigations have been developed. Another innovation has been the introduction of 'keyhole' surgery using an endoscope attached to a video camera. The avoidance of a large incision reduces postoperative pain and shortens the recovery period, but often prolongs the operation.

It was soon realized that a general anaesthetic was no longer required for all these procedures, and that most of the investigations could be performed under sedation, augmented, if necessary, with a topical or local anaesthetic. Many different techniques are now available, but most utilize an intravenous injection of a benzodiazepene drug such as diazepam, together with an analgesic such as pethidine. The patient becomes drowsy, but retains consciousness and can cooperate with the endoscopist. There is little memory of the unpleasant sensations associated with the procedure, because of the nature of the drug. Providing that the operator and assistant are properly trained, that appropriate monitoring is used, that recovery is carefully supervised, and that the patient does not drive or use machinery during the ensuing 24 hours, the procedure is remarkably satisfactory.

Sedation is also widely used when operations are performed under local, regional, spinal or epidural analgesia. The patient often sleeps and has no memory of the procedure, but can be awakened at will. Sedation techniques have also proved popular in dentistry, since they enable the dentist to treat patients who would otherwise refuse to attend because of fear.

Day-case or ambulatory surgery

The origins

Day-case surgery started in the Royal Hospital for Sick Children in Glasgow, Scotland. It was there that a paediatric surgeon, James Nicholl, realized that most children hate being admitted to hospital, and so started to operate on them as outpatients. In 1909, he reported not only that nearly 9000 operations had been carried out as day cases over a 10-year period, but also that he had secured accommodation close to the hospital so that nursing mothers could stay with their children while they were in hospital.[1] It was a remarkable achievement in such a poverty-stricken environment.

Another person who realized the advantages of day-case surgery was the anaesthetist Ralph Waters. He opened the so-called 'Downtown Anesthesia Clinic' in Sioux City, Iowa, in 1916.[2] This was described in Chapter 4. The surgery was limited to operations that could be carried out under nitrous oxide anaesthesia, although this agent was occasionally augmented by an opiate premedication. Stronger agents, such as ether, were rarely used, since they would have resulted in prolonged recovery and, often, postoperative vomiting. Surgical procedures were usually short – dental extractions, circumcisions, simple fractures or incision of abscesses – and patients were usually fit to go home within an hour or so. The success of the clinic was probably largely due to the fact that Waters was a very skilled anaesthetist who could manage to produce satisfactory operating conditions with this relatively weak but short-acting anaesthetic agent. But of equal importance was the fact that the patient and surgeon could book a mutually convenient time for the operation, and that costs were much less than inpatient treatment because of the lower overheads and the elimination of the overnight hospital stay.

Limitations of nitrous oxide

The failure to develop this idea in either the USA or UK over the next 30–40 years was probably due to the difficulties in achieving an adequate depth of anaesthesia with nitrous oxide–oxygen mixtures. These difficulties did not, however, deter British dentists from using nitrous oxide as the sole anaesthetic for extractions in the dental chair; it was quick and relatively safe and could be administered by another dentist. Although there were a few anaesthetists such as Robert Macintosh

(Chapter 5) who specialized in dental anaesthesia, most dental gases were given by general practitioners, who found that the modest fees provided a useful addition to their income.

It was, however, a rather terrifying procedure for all concerned. In some dental hospital clinics, 20–30 patients would be anaesthetized in a single three-hour session. The patient was strapped into the chair in the upright position and a mouth gag inserted to hold the mouth open. 100% nitrous oxide was then given through a nasal mask and a small percentage of oxygen added when the patient became cyanosed and unconscious. The dentist extracted the teeth as rapidly as possible and the anaesthetic was then discontinued, the whole procedure from induction to recovery usually being completed within a few minutes. Many patients did not like the smell of the mask or the gas, and they sometimes struggled violently as they passed through the stage of excitement into surgical anaesthesia, forcible restraint often being required when hard-drinking or belligerent males submitted themselves for extractions. Many patients experienced unpleasant dreams, and they often cried or laughed uncontrollably as they regained consciousness. Gas sessions in a children's hospital were rendered even more unpleasant by the screams of the young children undergoing this ordeal.

In some cases, recovery was prolonged, and a number of anaesthetists began to suspect that the brain had suffered hypoxic damage. In 1938–39, the American neuropathologist CB Courville described a series of patients who had suffered irreparable brain damage after the use of the secondary saturation technique of nitrous oxide administration.[3] This technique had been developed by EI McKesson in Toledo, Ohio in the 1920s in an attempt to produce abdominal relaxation for abdominal surgery, and, since it relied on severe hypoxia to relax the abdominal muscles, it was the subject of much controversy at the time.[4] The significance of Courville's studies did not become apparent to most British anaesthetists until after the war, but from the 1950s onwards, they attempted to avoid hypoxic damage by adding trichloroethylene (Trilene) to the gas mixture or by using a volatile agent such as divinyl ether (Vinesthene) when anaesthetizing children. Others began to use intravenous induction with thiopental, but this increased the risk of hypotension and also prolonged recovery. Since the only monitoring used in the dental chair was a finger on the pulse, the occurrence of hypotension was sometimes missed, with disastrous results.

In the 1960s, the new generation of anaesthetists began to recognize that general anaesthesia in the dental chair could result in hypotension and hypoxia, and that the procedure carried an unacceptable risk, so they began to campaign for a change in practice. It was not until the 1990s, however, that it was finally agreed that general anaesthesia would only be permitted in the dental surgery if the surgery was equipped to the same standard as the hospital operating suite. Since few dental surgeons could justify such an expense, most dental surgery is now performed under local anaesthesia with or without sedation, and patients requiring general anaesthesia are given a standard general anaesthetic in a hospital. There are, however, still some dental surgeons who adhere to the old practices, and this has prompted the Royal College of Anaesthetists to express its concerns about the use of general anaesthesia and sedation in the dental surgery.[5]

Ambulatory care

Throughout the first half of the 20th century, it was common to administer short general anaesthetics for surgical procedures such as myringotomy, reduction of fractures or incision of abscesses in the casualty department of the local hospital. Because the operation was brief and could be performed under a light anaesthetic, patients were often allowed to leave hospital after an hour or so. In the USA, similar procedures were often carried out in the doctor's office, but these constituted a small percentage of the surgical throughput. The difference between these practices and today's ambulatory surgery is that the surgery now takes place in a dedicated unit that is designed to enable a much wider range of surgical procedures to be carried out safely and expeditiously with a minimal duration of patient stay. The success of these units is largely due to the introduction of new short-acting intravenous and inhalation anaesthetic agents over the last half-century.

The first units

One of the first ambulatory surgical units was based in a hospital attached to the University of California, Los Angeles, and was described in 1962. Similar facilities were soon opened in other hospitals, and in 1969 a successful 'free-standing' unit was opened in Phoenix, Arizona. The initial growth of ambulatory surgery in the USA was due to the efforts of the private medical insurance groups to curb the escalating costs of surgical procedures, but in Europe, where healthcare provision is more state-orientated, there has been less incentive to develop such initiatives.[6] The result is that, whereas in the USA in 1994 over 60% of all surgical procedures were performed on an ambulatory basis, in the UK the figure was around 20%. However, the Department of Health's NHS Plan (2000) set a target that 75% of elective admissions should be operated on as day cases.[7]

The day case unit

In the UK, the ambulatory unit is usually part of a hospital, but often has a separate entrance. It contains a reception area, one or more operating theatres, and a recovery area. The key requirement is that the patient should not be suffering from a disease that would increase the risk of this type of treatment, and that there should be suitable homecare. The choice between standard or day-case treatment is usually made during the outpatient consultation. The second requirement is that the staff should be experienced and should work as an efficient team. Since anaesthetists have taken increasing responsibility for the running of main operating theatre suites, and since anaesthesia plays such a key role in ambulatory surgery, many of these units are now run by anaesthetists.

Advantages and disadvantages

There are major advantages for the patient: there is a defined date for the operation, and the operation is unlikely to be cancelled because of bed shortages or emergency admissions. Furthermore, the patient spends the minimum time away from the home environment and is less likely to acquire a hospital-based infection. The disadvantages are that the patient may suffer postoperative nausea, vomiting, discomfort or pain that may be exacerbated by the journey home, and there may be difficulty in obtaining medical or nursing help in the relatively rare event that complications develop later. Doctors running day-case units are fully aware of these problems, and take special precautions to avoid them. Most patients feel that the advantages far outweigh the possible disadvantages.[8]

The role of the anaesthetist

One of the major reasons why these units could be introduced in the 1960s and 70s was that three new non-explosive inhalation anaesthetic agents were introduced during this period: halothane (Fluothane), enflurane (Ethrane) and isoflurane (Forane). These agents were potent, relatively non-irritant to the airways and relatively insoluble in blood – properties that meant that a satisfactory depth of anaesthesia could be produced quickly and without coughing, and that recovery was equally speedy. Fortunately, the use of these new agents was also associated with a relatively low incidence of postoperative nausea and vomiting. In the last few years, two other volatile agents – sevoflurane and desflurane – with even shorter induction and recovery times have been introduced.

In the same period, a number of short-acting intravenous induction agents were being marketed. These drugs were designed to have a shorter action than thiopental (Pentothal) to avoid the somnolence that often followed a thiopental anaesthetic. However, all the intravenous drugs introduced in the 1960s and 70s have now been displaced by the latest intravenous anaesthetic, propofol (Diprivan), which has such a short duration of action that it can be given either as a single-shot induction agent or as a continuous infusion. The latter technique enables the anaesthetist to adjust the depth of anaesthesia to match the intensity of stimuli produced by the different stages of the surgery, and yet to have the patient awake and alert within a few minutes of the end of the operation.

Other short-acting drugs have helped the anaesthetist to develop minute-by-minute control of anaesthetic depth. For example, analgesic drugs such as fentanyl, alfentanil and remifentanil have largely displaced morphine and pethidine as intravenous supplements to nitrous oxide. Manufacturers have also marketed relatively short-acting synthetic muscle-relaxant drugs to replace the old faithful, curare, so now anaesthetists are able to speed up both the induction and recovery from anaesthesia and yet provide a perfect level of anaesthesia for any surgical procedure. It is the skilful use of these short-acting drugs, with or without regional anaesthesia with a local anaesthetic drug, that has enabled surgeons to extend the range of operations that can be performed in an ambulatory unit setting.

While the introduction of new short-acting drugs has been an important factor in the development of day-case surgery, we must also remember that the successful application of these drugs has been dependent on extensive human studies performed by anaesthetists and pharmacologists. Pharmacokinetic studies have shown how these drugs are distributed within the body tissues and how they are then metabolized and excreted, while pharmacodynamic studies have helped us to understand the way in which drugs act on cells to produce their effects. This kind of research has helped to define dosage schedules for continuous infusion, and has also shown how the drug profile may be modified by disease.

The future

In the 1950s, approximately three million anaesthetics were given in UK dental surgeries each year, but most of the patients who received an anaesthetic for other types of surgery had to remain in hospital overnight to recover from the anaesthetic. Today, general anaesthetics are rarely given in dental surgeries, but over 60% of patients undergoing other types of surgery are operated on as day cases, although there is a great variation between Hospital Trusts and between surgical specialities. The contrast between the pandemonium in the dental clinic of the 1950s and the peaceful environment of today's day-case units could not be greater.

With the increasing use of 'keyhole' surgical techniques, and the pressure on inpatient beds, it seems likely that day-case surgery will continue to expand. Patients like it, doctors and nurses like it, and administrators like it even more. But patients often ask 'Is day-case surgery safe?' The answer is that all the prerequisites for safety are built in to the selection process: a non-emergency, short operation with minimal blood loss; a fit patient; and experienced medical and nursing staff. The difficulty is to persuade everyone working in the hospital service that day-case surgery should be used more effectively.[9]

References

1. Nicoll JH. The surgery of infancy. *British Medical Journal* 1909:**ii**:753–4.
2. Waters RM. The down-town anesthesia clinic. *American Journal of Surgery (Anesthesia supplement)* 1919;**33**:71–3.
3. Courville CB. *Untoward Effects of Nitrous Oxide Anesthesia.* Mountain View, CA: Pacific Press Publishing Association, 1939.
4. Clement FW. *Nitrous-Oxide–Oxygen Anesthesia.* London: Henry Kimpton, 1939.
5. *Standards and Guidelines for General Anaesthesia for Dentistry*, London: Royal College of Anaesthetists, 1999.
6. Prabhu A, Chung F. Anaesthetic strategies towards developments in day care surgery. *European Journal of Anaesthesiology* 2001; **23**(Suppl):36–42.
7. *The NHS Plan.* London: Department of Health, 2000.
8. Twersky RS. Ambulatory surgery update. *Canadian Journal of Anaesthesia* 1998;**45**:76–90.
9. *Acute Hospital Portfolio Review: Day Surgery.* London: Healthcare Commission, 2005.

Part 4

The relief of pain in childbirth and the care of the newborn

From the earliest times until the 17th century, childbirth remained the province of the midwife or the female members of the family. Then, a few doctors began to specialize in the subject and developed operative techniques for dealing with obstetric complications. James Young Simpson in Edinburgh was the first to use the newly discovered ether analgesia and anaesthesia to relieve the pain of labour, and within a year he had also introduced chloroform into obstetric practice.

In the 1930s, the anaesthetist RJ Minnitt in Liverpool developed a machine for delivering a fixed mixture of nitrous oxide and air that could be used by midwives to alleviate the pains of labour when a doctor was not present; in the 1950s, trichloroethylene inhalers were developed for the same purpose. In the late 1940s in the USA, RA Hingson popularized the use of epidural anaesthesia given by an injection into the base of the spine, while in the UK, other anaesthetists began to use epidural analgesia given by the lumbar route. The role of midwives varies between countries, but their views have important implications for the delivery of obstetric pain relief, and there is still an ongoing debate about the use of epidural analgesia in labour. The use of these new methods of pain relief has had a major impact on childbirth throughout the developed world. We deal first with the problem of relieving pain in normal labour and then discuss anaesthesia for operative obstetrics. Finally, we tell the story of Virginia Apgar, a remarkable anesthesiologist who evolved a scoring system for assessing the baby's condition at birth. The Apgar score is now used worldwide to predict the need for resuscitation of the newborn baby.

20 Pain relief for the woman in labour

'Man endures pain as an undeserved punishment; woman accepts it as a natural heritage' (**Anonymous**)

The use of inhalational agents

At the Royal Infirmary in Edinburgh, on 19 January 1847, less than three months after Morton's successful demonstration of ether anaesthesia in Boston, James Young Simpson administered ether to an unidentified woman to relieve the pain of a difficult delivery. It is the first recorded administration of an anaesthetic to relieve the pain of labour.[1] The first woman in America to receive anaesthesia to relieve the pain of labour, this time for a normal delivery, was the wife of a very famous poet. The date was 7 April 1847, the patient Fanny Appleton Longfellow, wife of Henry Wadsworth Longfellow, and the anaesthetist Nathan Cooley Keep.[2] Keep was a distinguished doctor and dentist who later became the first Dean of Harvard Dental School. Describing the occasion Longfellow wrote:

> *'Fanny heroically inhaled the vapor of sulfuric ether, the great nepenthe, and all of the pain of labor ceased, though the labor itself went on and seemed accelerated. This is the first trial of ether at such time in this country. It has been completely successful. While under the influence of the vapor, there was no loss of consciousness, but no pain. All ended happily'.*[3]

Backed by his prestige as Professor of Midwifery at the University of Edinburgh, Simpson set about championing the use of ether in childbirth; he was joined in this endeavour by the Professor of Midwifery and Jurisprudence at Harvard University, Walter Channing.[4] Despite the imprimatur of such distinguished doctors and the institutions they represented, there was widespread opposition from medical practitioners, just as there had been to anaesthesia in surgery. Pain, it was believed, was necessary part of the normal process of birth. Leading the opposition to anaesthesia was the Philadelphia obstetrician Charles Meigs, who wrote of the morally '*doubtful nature of any process that the physicians set up to contravene the operation of those natural and physiological factors that the Divinity has ordained us to enjoy or to suffer*'.[5] Joining forces in united opposition, the Church of England objected on moral and scriptural grounds, quoting the Bible's admonition to Eve that 'in sorrow thou shalt bring forth children' (Genesis 3, v. 16). Brushing aside such theological objections, Simpson called again on the authority of the Bible to claim that the good book sanctioned anaesthesia: '. . . *the Lord God caused a deep sleep to fall upon Adam, and he slept; and he took one of his ribs and closed the flesh, thereof*' (Genesis 2, v. 21), thus anaesthetizing Adam for the delivery of Eve; Simpson also pointed out that, while the Bible admonished Eve to bring forth children in sorrow, the word 'sorrow' in Hebrew meant 'to work' as well as 'to suffer', that a woman must work during the birth of a child, but not necessarily experience pain.[6,7]

Theological objections aside, doctors – again not unreasonably – worried about the possibility of anaesthetic fatalities during labour. The administration of ether in labour had been largely supplanted by chloroform, less irritant than ether but a more potent and an inherently more dangerous agent.[8] Thomas Wakley, editor of *The Lancet*, on learning that Queen Victoria might have received chloroform during the birth of her eighth child, Prince Leopold, on 7 April 1853, wrote in dismay that chloroform is '*an agent which has unquestionably caused instantaneous death in a considerable number of cases*'.[9] Although Wakley chose to disbelieve that doctors had allowed the Queen to inhale chloroform, it was the Queen herself who had made the decision, with the pronouncement that '*We are going to have this baby, and We are going to have chloroform.*' John Snow, famous for halting the waterborne epidemic of cholera in London a year later, was her anaesthetist (Figure 20.1). He sprinkled chloroform onto a handkerchief so that it was inhaled in low concentration with each contraction. This provided pain relief without actual loss of consciousness. Describing the experience later, the Queen wrote that Snow '*gave that blessed chloroform and the effect was soothing, quieting & delightful beyond measure*'. Four years later, she received chloroform anaesthesia again on the birth of Princess Beatrice. '*Anésthésie a la reine*', as it soon was known, became fashionable, and objections gradually faded away.[10,11]

During the remainder of the 19th century, there were sporadic attempts to relieve pain in labour by means other than inhalation anaesthetics.

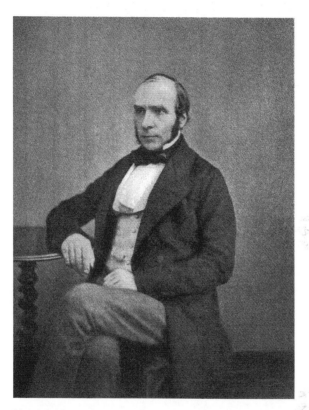

Figure 20.1 John Snow (1813–1858), who administered chloroform to Queen Victoria for the birth of two of her children. Snow was the first anaesthetist to apply science to anaesthesia. He was also famous for his studies of cholera epidemics and terminated a London epidemic by removing the handle of the Broad Street pump. (Reproduced with permission from the Association of Anaesthetists of Great Britain and Ireland.)

These included morphine and morphine-like drugs, and the rectal administration of chloral hydrate or ether dissolved in oil, but these drugs all depressed the fetal respiratory centre and resulted in delayed onset of breathing after birth.

Injection of pain-relieving drugs

Next in the search for pain-free labour was 'Dammerschlaf', or twilight sleep, introduced in Austria in 1902. The woman in labour received injections of morphine to provide initial pain relief, followed by hyoscine (scopolamine) to provide sedation and loss of memory of pain. Further injections of hyoscine prolonged the loss of consciousness. It was claimed that with this technique the woman had no memory of the delivery and that there was no harm to the baby. The technique became popular with obstetricians, but patients needed to be restrained by straps to prevent them falling out of bed during their semicomatose state. It eventually became clear that this technique was associated with prolongation of labour and an increase in infant mortality due to respiratory depression. Despite these disadvantages, twilight sleep continued to be used in America until the mid-20th century.

Self-administered analgesia

From the 1930s onwards, the methods of pain control in the UK and in the USA differed because of differences in obstetric staffing. In the UK, the tradition of delivery by midwives remained strong, and many deliveries were carried out by certified midwives without doctors being present, but in the USA, deliveries had increasingly become the responsibility of doctors, and midwives were limited to remote or poverty-stricken communities. In her book *The American Way of Birth*, Jessica Mitford argued that this state of affairs was largely engineered by greedy doctors, but the obstetricians claimed that they could provide a safer environment than the midwife.[12] In the UK, the percentage of deliveries in hospital has gradually increased, so that only about 2% of deliveries now take place in the home. However, midwives still deliver about 50% of normal births. This has led to the development of methods of analgesia that can be used by midwives when a doctor is not present, either at home or in hospital.

One of the first to introduce such a method was RJ Minnitt, an anaesthetist in Liverpool.[13] He devised a simple apparatus delivering a fixed mixture of 35% nitrous oxide in air; equipped with a face mask, the woman in labour could then 'self-administer' the mixture with each contraction (Figures 20.2 and 20.3). The apparatus was approved for use by the mother under midwife supervision in 1936. It was a small step forward in that some pain relief was obtained. But when nitrous oxide was added to room air, inhaled oxygen was decreased proportionately. This, in turn, lowered the amount of oxygen received by the baby, potentially compromising the baby's survival. The technique was largely abandoned in the 1950s when the apparatus was found to malfunction, and from 1970 onward midwives were not allowed to use a gas/air mixture.

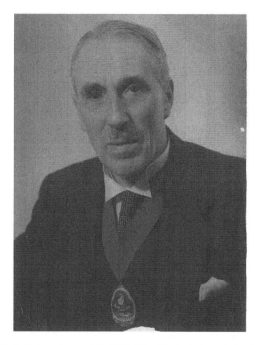

Figure 20.2 Dr Robert James Minnitt (1899–1974) of Liverpool, who, in 1933, pioneered the use of nitrous oxide to relieve the pain of childbirth. (Reproduced by kind permission of the University of Liverpool Department of Anaesthesia.)

In 1941, trichloroethylene (Trilene) was introduced into British anaesthetic practice. Originally used as a degreasing agent in industry, it was later found that its inhalation diminished the pain of trigeminal neuralgia ('tic douloureux'). When inhaled in a concentration of 0.35–0.5% it provided better pain relief than nitrous oxide, without loss of consciousness. It was administered by specially designed vaporizers, and was approved for use by midwives in 1954 (Figure 20.4). Midwives were also licensed to administer limited doses of what was then a new synthetic narcotic, pethidine (meperidine; Demerol). If administered in limited dosage, pethidine did not appear to depress the newborn baby's respiration, but many patients complained that it did not give pain relief either.

Although machines delivering fixed concentrations of nitrous oxide in oxygen were developed, they were soon made redundant by the

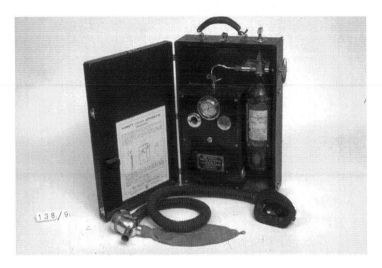

Figure 20.3 The Minnitt gas and air apparatus that was licensed for use by midwives in the absence of a doctor. The metal CM attachment could be added to the breathing system if a doctor was present. This enabled the patient to breath a limited quantity of 100% nitrous oxide from the bag, thus speeding up the onset of analgesia. When the bag emptied, the patient received the gas and air mixture. (Nuffield Department of Anaesthetics, Oxford.)

introduction of 50/50 nitrous oxide/oxygen mixtures stored in gas cylinders.[14] The mixture was introduced into clinical practice in 1961, and in 1965 it was approved for use under midwife supervision. The mixture, known as Entonox, is now piped into most obstetrical units so that it is available beside each delivery ward bed. Since it is not only an effective analgesic but also enriches the oxygen supply to mother and baby, it has now largely displaced other inhalation agents in labour. Entonox is also used in accident and emergency departments, intensive care units, and paramedic ambulances to provide short-term pain relief.

Regional analgesia

Today, the most popular method of pain relief during labour is provided by epidural anaesthesia, the injection of local anaesthetic drugs that block the nerves as they leave the dura mater, which encloses the cerebrospinal fluid and spinal cord. This results in anaesthesia of the lower part of the body. The controversy over the administration of this

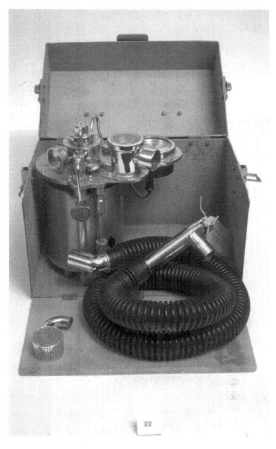

Figure 20.4 The EMOTRIL (Epstein–Macintosh–Oxford–Trilene) inhaler, one of three trichloroethylene (Trilene) inhalers certified for use by midwives in the absence of a doctor. (Nuffield Department of Anaesthetics, Oxford.)

form of anaesthesia in obstetrics is not unlike that of a 150 years ago. It again centres on whether pain relief is achieved at the expense of interference with a normal and essential biological process. Is the pain of uterine contraction essential to safe delivery and to optimal fetal and maternal health, and to what extent does the administration of epidural anaesthesia interfere with this essential process? Opposing the routine use of epidural anaesthetics in normal and low-risk vaginal delivery are the midwives, on whom the responsibility for care during labour ordinarily falls. They believe that *'women want woman-centred care, that they want continuity of care, and that they want childbirth to be seen as a physiological, not as a pathological process, whenever possible'*. They argue that the need for analgesia is markedly reduced when one-to-one care is provided by a trained nurse–midwife (a claim that remains to be substantiated). They also point out that, with epidural anaesthesia, labour may be prolonged, that instrumental delivery is more apt to be necessary, and that there is a small increase in the frequency of complications (although almost all of these are relatively minor).[15]

Against these drawbacks, epidural anaesthesia provides reliable pain relief in all but a small number of cases. In the contemporary environment in which patients are better informed and can choose the treatment they wish to receive, many women opt for the pain relief that epidural anaesthesia can provide. Many do not, however. Among women who had declined pain relief during labour, reasons given included the belief that *'pain is an integral part of the childbirth experience'*, that they *'want to experience birth for its own sake'*, that they felt the *'need to stay in control'*, and that *'pain brings its own rewards'*.[16] Among 100 women undergoing vaginal delivery at Queen Charlotte's Maternity Hospital in London who were given a choice of method of pain relief, just over half chose epidural anaesthesia. Questioned 48 hours following delivery, *'there were more dissatisfied women among the epidural patients than among those who did not receive this analgesia'*. Interviewed a year later, their 'bad experience' was associated with forceps delivery and prolonged labour, each of which were more common in women who had received epidural anaesthesia.[17]

Regional anaesthetic techniques used in labour today are, however, very different from those used in the 1970s and 80s. The addition of opioid drugs such as fentanyl to the local anaesthetic solution allows more dilute concentrations of local anaesthetic to be used. This enables the anaesthetist to abolish the pain of labour without also paralysing the muscles (the so-called 'walking epidural'), so the woman can retain more control over the birth process. Another technique, the combined spinal–epidural, utilizes injections into the spinal fluid and epidural space, thus enabling the anaesthetist to utilize the advantages of both techniques.[18]

When anaesthetists started to provide an epidural service in the 1960s, they had to combine this work with many other commitments, so they started to teach midwives to give supplementary doses of local anaesthetic via the epidural catheter and to remove the catheter after delivery. The constraints on the doctor's time limited the number of epidurals that could be performed, and such a service could only be provided in a limited number of centres. In the 1970s and 80s, obstetric anaesthesia services in the UK were gradually reorganized so that obstetric units were staffed by Consultants and juniors throughout 24 hours. This has enabled an epidural service to be provided in the majority of hospitals with maternity units, and has done much to improve the standard of obstetric analgesia. It has, however, had major staffing and financial implications.

The problem of pain relief during normal labour is of obvious concern to the mother and her attendants, but the provision of anaesthesia for operative obstetrics is a very different problem, since the mother's life is at stake. As we shall see in the next chapter, the risks of anaesthesia are now very much less than they were 50 years ago.

References

1. Simpson JY. Notes on the employment of the inhalation of sulphuric ether in the practice of midwifery. *Monthly Journal of Medical Sciences* 1847/48;**7**:721–8.
2. Keep NC. The letheon administered in a case of labor. *Boston Medical and Surgical Journal* 1847;**36**:226.
3. Longfellow HW. *Journal,1847–1848.* Quoted by Pittinger CB. The anesthetization of Fanny Longfellow for childbirth on April 7, 1847. *Anesthesia and Analgesia* 1987;**66**:368–9.
4. Channing WA. *A Treatise on Etherization in Childbirth.* Boston: Ticknor, 1848.
5. Meigs CD. *Females and Their Diseases.* Philadelphia: Lea and Blanchard, 1848.
6. Simpson JY. *Answer to Religious Objections Advanced Against the Employment of Anaesthetic Agents in Midwifery and Surgery.* Edinburgh: Sutherland and Knox, 1847.
7. Farr AD. Early opposition to obstetric anaesthesia. *Anaesthesia* 1980;**35**:896–907.
8. Simpson JY. An account of a new anaesthetic agent as a substitute for sulphuric ether in surgery and midwifery. *Medico-Chirurgical Society of Edinburgh.* 12 November 1847.
9. Wakley T. Leading article. *Lancet* 14 May 1853. Quoted in Sykes WS. *Essays on the First Hundred Years of Anaesthesia.* Vol. 1. Huntington, NY: Robert E Krieger, 1972: 79.
10. Poppers PJ. The history and development of obstetric anesthesia. In: Rupreht J, van Lieburg MJ, Lee JA, Erdmann W, eds. *Anaesthesia: Essays on its History.* Berlin: Springer-Verlag, 1985: 133–40.
11. Russell CA. Objections to anaesthesia: the case of James Young Simpson. In: Smith EB, Daniels S, eds. *Gases in Medicine: Anaesthesia.* Cambridge: Royal Society of Chemistry, 1998: 173–87.
12. Mitford J. *The American Way of Birth.* London: Victor Gollancz, 1992.
13. Minnitt RJ. Self-administered analgesia for the midwifery of general practice. *Proceedings of the Royal Society of Medicine* 1934;**27**:1313–18.

14. Tunstall ME. Obstetric anaesthesia. The use of a fixed nitrous oxide and oxygen mixture from one cylinder. *Lancet* 1961;**ii**:964.
15. Brighouse D. Epidural analgesia in labour is not compatible with midwife-led care. *International Journal of Obstetric Anesthesia* 1996;**5**:126–9.
16. Jowitt M. Pain in labour – is it insufferable?: mothers' experience and attitudes. *Midwifery Matters* Summer 2000.
17. Morgan BM, Bulpitt CJ, Clifton P, Lewis PJ. Analgesia and satisfaction in childbirth (the Queen Charlotte's 1000 Mother Survey). *Lancet* 1982;**ii**:808–10.
18. Comparative Obstetric Mobile Epidural Trial (COMET) Study Group UK. Randomized controlled trial comparing traditional with two 'mobile' epidural techniques. *Anesthesiology* 2002;**97**:1567–75.

21 Anaesthesia for obstetric procedures in the UK

In the UK in the 1950s, about 50% of women were delivered at home.[1] When complications set in, there was usually no time to transfer the patient to hospital, so the 'flying squad' was called out. The junior anaesthetist was part of the team, and was often as frightened as the patient. Now only about 2% of women are delivered at home, and most women have the chance of choosing whether they wish to be awake or asleep during the delivery of their baby.

The 'flying squad'

The 'flying squad' was a hospital-based team consisting of a resident obstetrician, anaesthetist and midwife who could be called out by the district midwife if she encountered difficulties with a home delivery. When the call came, we rushed down to the casualty department, picked up the basket containing the instruments, transfusion apparatus, and bottles of plasma and blood, and roared out into the night in an ambulance. Sometimes, the mother's condition permitted transfer to hospital – but not infrequently she needed resuscitation with fluid and blood and immediate instrumental delivery, since delay would have greatly increased the risk to mother or baby.

The conditions in the home were usually appalling. The mother would be lying in a soaking wet bed with the family around, and she would probably have had a meal of fish and chips. The only anaesthetic agents that could be transported easily were chloroform and ether, and the latter could not be administered if there was a fire in the room because of the risk of explosion. Most junior anaesthetists had not been taught how to use open-drop chloroform, and it was not easy to hold up the chin, control the rate at which the drops were falling onto the mask, monitor the pulse and respiration, and control the blood transfusion while kneeling on a flimsy mattress. Meanwhile, the obstetrician would be tugging on the forceps or performing some other obstetric manoeuvre in an attempt to deliver a live baby. In those days, the blood transfusion was delivered through stiff red rubber tubing attached to a large, sharp intravenous needle, so it was difficult to prevent the tip cutting through the vein wall while the patient was being pulled around the bed. Fortunately, less than 2% of births now occur in the home, and the 'flying squads' no longer exist.

But emergencies still occur in hospital practice. When the birth is complicated by some obstetric complication such as a breech presentation or disproportion, it may be necessary to turn the baby into the head-down position, or apply forceps. It may even be necessary to deliver the baby by Caesarean section: in some centres, 20–30% of all babies are born in this way. An anaesthetic may also be required if the patient bleeds from an abnormally placed placenta, or when the placenta fails to separate after birth. The real emergency, however, is the occurrence of fetal distress due to obstruction of the umbilical cord or to placental insufficiency. Whatever the reason for the anaesthetic, the anaesthetist must always remember that there are two patients – the mother and the baby – and, since many drugs cross the placenta, general anaesthesia for the mother invariably results in depressed respiration in the baby.

If an epidural catheter is already in place, the anaesthetist may be able to extend the block to provide sufficient anaesthesia for the procedure. Sometimes, a spinal anaesthetic may be used, but if regional anaesthesia is not possible, the anaesthetist will give a general anaesthetic. Unfortunately, each of these techniques brings its own set of problems. Some of the problems associated with spinals and epidurals have already been discussed, but the problems of general anaesthesia are even greater.

General anaesthesia

The mother undergoes many anatomical, physiological and hormonal changes during pregnancy, and these may cause problems for the anaesthetist. For example, if the mother lies supine, the weight of the baby may obstruct the inferior vena cava and so cause circulatory collapse. To prevent this, the mother lies on her side. This increases the difficulty of tracheal intubation, a manoeuvre that is already rendered difficult by swelling of the tongue due to the fluid retention associated with pregnancy.

The passage of a cuffed tube is highly desirable, since the large uterus increases the pressure within the abdomen and so tends to cause regurgitation of fluid into the pharynx. If this acid fluid is aspirated into the lungs, it can produce Mendelson's syndrome, a particularly severe reaction in the lung tissue that often proves fatal. The risk of aspiration is greatest at induction of anaesthesia, so special precautions have to be taken to minimize the risk to the mother. In addition to a restricted food and fluid intake, an antacid is administered before induction of anaesthesia. The anaesthetist will then instruct an assistant to perform Sellick's manoeuvre just as the patient drifts off to sleep.

Brian Sellick was a Consultant Anaesthetist at the Middlesex Hospital in London who studied the problem of aspiration of stomach contents into the lungs (Figure 21.1). In 1961, he demonstrated that firm backward

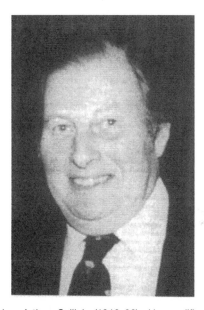

Figure 21.1 Brian Arthur Sellick (1918–96). He qualified in 1941, was appointed Resident Anaesthetist to the Middlesex Hospital, London, and gave most of the anaesthetics for emergency surgery during the Blitz. He then served as a specialist anaesthetist in the Royal Naval Volunteer Reserve in Australia and the Far East, and was appointed Consultant to the Middlesex Hospital in 1946. He and the surgeon Thomas Holmes Sellors visited Henry Swan's cardiac surgery clinic in Denver, Colorado in 1956 and successfully introduced Swan's technique of surface cooling for cardiac surgery. In 1961, Sellick visited the Mayo Clinic and supervised the introduction and use of the heart–lung machine in several London Hospitals. He described the manoeuvre that bears his name in 1961. (Reproduced with kind permission from Pallister WK. Brian Arthur Sellick. *Anaesthesia* 1996;**51**:1194–5.)

pressure on the cricoid cartilage could occlude the oesophagus and thus prevent regurgitation from the stomach.[2] This pressure has to be applied just as the patient goes to sleep, and then maintained until the tube is in place and the cuff inflated. This brilliant solution to the problem of aspiration and the adoption of a 'failed intubation drill' has undoubtedly been responsible for a reduction in deaths due to general anaesthesia in labour. It is of interest that both Charles Kite in London and James Curry in Northampton had advocated the use of a technique similar to that proposed by Sellick in the late 18th century, but they were attempting to prevent overdistension of the stomach during mouth-to-mouth ventilation.[3,4]

Another major problem is that any anaesthetic given to the mother also tends to pass through the placenta to the baby. Since many of the drugs used during anaesthesia depress respiration, the baby may not breathe adequately at birth. For this reason, the anaesthetist has to keep the mother in the lightest possible level of anaesthesia until the baby has been delivered. Unfortunately, this increases the risk that the mother may regain consciousness and possibly suffer pain during the procedure. This is a rare event, but is extremely distressing for the patient.

Recent progress

Obstetric anaesthesia has undergone vast changes over the past half-century. In the 1950s, there were only a few anaesthetists who devoted most of their time to obstetric problems. Midwives took care of pain relief, and the anaesthetist was only called to the labour ward when there was an obstetric emergency. The resident anaesthetist was often inexperienced and frequently involved with an emergency elsewhere in the hospital. By the time the anaesthetist had reached the labour ward, the patient was often in a critical condition. The anaesthetist would be in unfamiliar surroundings and would have no assistance, because the midwives were helping the obstetrician. The anaesthetist would have to check the anaesthetic machine, probably replace empty gas cylinders, find and draw up the appropriate drugs, set up an intravenous infusion, and then administer the anaesthetic to a terrified woman who might have suffered catastrophic blood loss or might have a full stomach. If a paediatrician was not available, the anaesthetist would have to resuscitate the baby as well. It is small wonder that anaesthesia-related deaths occurred.

Nowadays, most anaesthetic departments provide a dedicated obstetric anaesthesia service throughout 24 hours. The responsibility for running the obstetric anaesthesia service is allocated to a number of consultants who are responsible for equipping and running the unit, training junior staff, and providing pain relief throughout labour. The tremendous improvements that that have been implemented in the last half-century were largely driven by the findings of the triennial Confidential Enquiries into Maternal Deaths. These regular reports have made a huge impact on patient safety.

The Confidential Enquiries

In the late 1920s it was noted that, whereas infant and adult mortality rates had been falling steadily during the early 20th century, maternal mortality remained high. Since this was a cause of great public concern, the Minister of Health appointed a Departmental Committee on Maternal Morbidity and Mortality. This presented an Interim Report in 1930 and a Final Report in 1932. The reports were based on information collected by Medical Officers of Health throughout England and Wales, and covered 5800 cases of maternal death. In these reports, the investigators endeavoured to identify a 'primary avoidable factor' in the circumstances of a maternal death – that is to say, a departure from generally accepted standards of care as they were at that time. They found that such a factor was present in 45.9% of the deaths investigated. Since the maternal death rate was 4.4 per 1000 total births, this meant that there was considered to be an avoidable cause of death in about 1350 of the 3000 deaths per annum recorded in these initial reports. The reports also highlighted a large number of other deficiencies in the obstetric service. The reports were considered to be so valuable that Medical Officers of Health were asked to continue submitting their reports to the Chief Medical Officer, who summarized the results in successive Annual Reports 'On the State of the Public Health'.

By 1951 the maternal mortality rate had fallen to 0.8 per 1000 total births, representing a total of 566 deaths per year. However, the proportion of deaths due to a primary avoidable factor had not changed, and the proportion of deaths that could be investigated had fallen to about 60% because the data collection system was no longer working effectively. It was therefore decided to set up a new system of reporting. The new system aimed to 'place the clinical enquiries and assessment of avoidable factors in the hands of practising consultant obstetricians'. Significantly for us, an anaesthetist was invited to join the central group of obstetric assessors to provide an expert opinion on deaths associated with anaesthesia.

In the first *Report on Confidential Enquiries into Maternal Deaths in England and Wales 1952–54*, there were 1094 deaths classified as being due to pregnancy or childbirth.[5] The major causes of death were toxaemia of pregnancy (22% of the total), haemorrhage (17%), abortion (14%) and pulmonary embolism (13%). These four conditions accounted for two-thirds of the deaths directly due to pregnancy and childbirth.

In the same period, there were 49 deaths considered to be due to the complications of anaesthesia, and a further 20 in which anaesthesia may have contributed to the fatal outcome. The most common cause of death in patients submitted to anaesthesia was inhalation of stomach contents. Six deaths occurred during the administration of chloroform, and in two cases the obstetrician had induced general anaesthesia and then handed over to a nurse while he applied forceps. This first report was published in 1957, and was followed by others that showed equally disturbing statistics. In 1951, the Association of Anaesthetists also highlighted the problem with a report of 43 cases of regurgitation or vomiting during anaesthesia that resulted in death.[6]

In each triennium from 1952 until 1981, there were between 30 and 50 deaths in England and Wales that were described as being directly due to anaesthesia. In 1982–84, there were 19 such deaths, and in the 12 years from 1985 to 1996, there were also 19 deaths. In the report for the triennium 1994–96 (which included England, Wales, Scotland and Northern Ireland), there was only 1 death directly due to anaesthesia.[7] This astonishing reduction in mortality due to anaesthesia was probably due to four factors: first, the recognition that general anaesthesia in the pregnant patient is associated with an increased risk of complications; second, the development of special techniques of anaesthesia, including the widespread adoption of cricoid pressure and a 'failed intubation drill' to deal with these problems; third, the development of dedicated anaesthesia services for obstetrics; and fourth, the widespread adoption of epidural analgesia both for pain relief in labour and for operative obstetrics. Unfortunately, recent reports have revealed a small increase in anaesthetic-related deaths.[8] These have tended to occur in isolated units where trainees have not had adequate supervision, and are a cause for concern.[9]

The provision of dedicated anaesthetic services for the obstetric department required a major allocation of resources from the National Health Service (NHS), and is another reason for the increase in the number of anaesthetists in the NHS. It was the evidence provided by the Association of Anaesthetists' study of anaesthetic deaths and successive Confidential Enquiries that precipitated the changes, but it was the combined efforts of the Royal College of Anaesthetists, the Association of Anaesthetists, the Obstetric Anaesthetists Association, and the many Consultants who accepted responsibility for the obstetric anaesthesia services that finally ensured that appropriate standards were achieved.

The problem today

The problem for anaesthetists today is that mothers have many different ideas about pain in the earlier stages of labour. Some prefer minimal interference in the hope that they can achieve a natural labour; others demand all the pain relief that the anaesthetist can provide. The good obstetric anaesthetist will understand that no mother can predict how she will respond to the pain of labour, and will provide psychological support and the appropriate form of pain relief when requested. It is, however, often difficult to resolve the conflicting viewpoints and ideologies of patients and midwives.

There is still a major debate about the role of pain relief in labour, many midwives and some mothers believing that epidural analgesia should be used less frequently. But there is also a major change in the practice of obstetrics. More mothers are delaying their childbearing to their late 30s, by which time complications of childbirth are more frequent, and the fear of litigation drives many obstetricians to opt for the more controllable method of delivery by Caesarean section. Fortunately, the new generation of obstetric anaesthetists are well aware of these concerns, and most try to discuss the various options with patients before the delivery. Further progress can only be made when the current litigious climate is dispelled by constructive discussion between patient, midwife and doctor.

We have so far concentrated our attention on the mother, but we must not forget the baby. As we have noted, the neonate is affected by anaesthetic drugs given to the mother, but it may also suffer because there is placental insufficiency or because there is an obstruction to blood flow through the umbilical cord. The next chapter tells us how Virginia Apgar solved the problem of assessing the baby's condition at birth. This was a key development in reducing fetal mortality.

References

1. Kitzinger S, quoted in Mitford S. *The American Way of Birth*. London: Victor Gollancz, 1992: 208.
2. Sellick BA. Cricoid pressure to control regurgitation of stomach contents during induction of anaesthesia: preliminary communication. *Lancet* 1961;**ii**:404–6.
3. Kite C. *An Essay on the Recovery of the Apparently Dead*. London: C Dilly, 1778.
4. Curry J. *Popular Observations on Apparent Death from Drowning,*

   Suffocation etc. With an Account of the Means to be Employed for Recovery.
   Northampton: T Dicey, 1792.
5. *A Report on Confidential Enquiries into Maternal Deaths in England and
   Wales in 1952–54. Ministry of Health: Reports on Public Health and Medical
   Subjects*, No. 97. London: Her Majesty's Stationery Office, 1957.
6. Morton HJV, Wylie WD. Anaesthetic deaths due to regurgitation or vomiting.
   Anaesthesia 1951;**6**:190–201.
7. *The Confidential Enquiries into Maternal Deaths in the United Kingdom
   1994–6.* London: The Stationery Office, 1998.
8. *Why Mothers Die 2000-2002: The Sixth Report of the Confidential Enquiry
   into Maternal Death in the United Kingdom.* London: RCOG Press, 2004.
9. Clyburn PA. Editorial 2. Early thoughts on 'Why mothers die 2000–2002'.
   Anaesthesia 2004;**59**:1155–9.

Further reading

Pater N, ed. *Maternal Mortality – The Way Forward. Some Implications of the
   Report on Confidential Enquiries into Maternal Deaths in the United Kingdom
   1985–7.* London: Royal College of Obstetricians and Gynaecologists, 1992.
Kee WDN. Editorial: Confidential Enquiries into Maternal Deaths: 50 years of
   closing the loop. *British Journal of Anaesthesia* 2005;**94**:413–16.

22 Virginia Apgar and the care of the newborn

Virginia Apgar was the first woman to be named a full professor in Columbia University College of Physicians and Surgeons, New York. She set new standards of care in obstetric anaesthesia and described a simple but effective way of assessing the condition of the infant at birth.

With the completion of childbirth, who undertakes the immediate responsibility for the newborn baby's welfare? Who will undertake resuscitation if the baby is unresponsive, apnoeic or blue? In a high-risk pregnancy in a hospital obstetrical suite, it will in most cases be a paediatrician, often one trained in neonatology. With an elective Caesarean section following a normal pregnancy, a paediatrician may or may not be in attendance, and in a vaginal delivery at the conclusion of a low-risk pregnancy it would be unusual for a paediatrician to be present. In the absence of the paediatrician, it may fall on the anaesthetist, the midwife or the obstetrician to resuscitate a depressed newborn infant. For this, the anaesthetist is often the best qualified.

Fifty years ago, there were no paediatric neonatologists. The obstetrician or midwife would have been busy attending to the mother, and it fell on the circulating nurse or, if in attendance, the anaesthetist to undertake resuscitation when needed. At the moment of birth, the initial and urgent task is to judge the baby's condition. There were at that time no clearly established criteria for making that judgement. Virginia Apgar, Professor of Obstetrical Anesthesia at Columbia University in New York City, set out to provide them (Figure 22.1). Here, according to legend, is how it began. At a hospital breakfast one morning, perhaps after a night of deliveries, a medical student asked her how one should evaluate the condition of a newborn baby, to which Apgar replied *'"That's easy! You'd do like this"* She grabbed the nearest piece of paper, jotted down

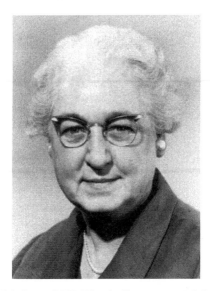

Figure 22.1 Virginia Apgar (1909–74) – the first woman at Columbia University College of Physicians and Surgeons to be named a full professor.

the five points of [what became known as] *the Apgar Score, then rushed off to the O.B (obstetric department) to try it out'.*[1]

The score that she proposed and published in 1953 consisted of five 'signs': heart rate, respiratory effort, reflex irritability, muscle tone and skin colour. Each sign was given a rating of 0, 1 or 2. For example, a heart rate of 100–140 beats/min was given a score of 2, a rate of under 100 beats/min a score of 1, and if no heartbeat could be detected the score was 0. Adding the five scores gave a total of 10 for a baby in the best possible condition. Scores of 8–10 indicate an infant in good condition, 4–7 the need for careful observation, and a score less than 4 the need for immediate resuscitative measures.[2] '*The score that she constructed*,' the Yale epidemiologist Alvin Feinstein later wrote, '*was a pioneer attempt to convert an intangible clinical phenomenon into a formally specified measurement*'.[3]

The time chosen to assign the score, after both the top of the head and bottoms of the feet were visible, was 60 seconds, the importance of which Apgar said could not be overestimated. Time, she knew from her years of experience, is of the essence and needed to be measured precisely, preferably with an automatic timer set to ring at 55 seconds, thus allowing 5 seconds, all that was considered necessary for the observation of the five signs. A 5-minute Apgar Score was added later and proved to provide important prognostic information, as discussed below.

Who is to assign the score? This was a matter of considerable importance. A paediatrician, if in attendance, can give full attention to the newborn baby's condition. The obstetrician or midwife will be fully occupied in the care of the mother. The circulating nurse will have a multiplicity of other duties at the time of birth, but may be the only professional present in addition to the obstetrician or midwife, and will be expected to attend to the baby. An anaesthetist, if in attendance, may be relatively free to observe the baby, to assign a score, and to respond quickly as the baby's condition requires. '*Only clinicians in anesthesia have learned to live by the second hand of a watch*,' Apgar wrote, '*To others, a minute is an unbelievably short interval*'.[4]

After its publication, the Apgar Score rapidly became the standard by which the condition of the newborn baby at the moment of birth was judged throughout the world. One- and five-minute scores have been included on the US Standard Certificate of Birth since 1978, and are published in the *US Annual National Vital Statistics Report*, together with birthweight and other statistics relating to childbearing. Since its publication, the Apgar Score has been cited in the medical literature three-quarters of a million times.

Today, in the words of an anonymous doctor, '*Every baby born in a modern hospital anywhere in the world is looked at first through the eyes of Virginia Apgar*.' APGAR became an acronym, the five signs reworded for easy memory as '**A**ppearance, **P**ulse, **G**rimace, **A**ctivity and **R**espiration'. Apgar became a legend in her lifetime, a legend memorialized in 1994 by inclusion in the US Postal Service Great American Series postage stamps (Figure 22.2).

Apgar's initial purpose was to establish a system to predict survival, to compare several methods of resuscitation that were in use, and:

> '... through the infant's responsiveness after delivery, to compare perinatal experience in different hospitals. The influence of various obstetrical practices such as the induction of labour, elective Caesarean section and maternal anaesthesia and analgesia might well be reflected in the score. It was furthermore hoped that the scoring system would ensure closer observation of the infant during the first minute of life'.[4]

The important use of the scoring system's potential in neonatal research became apparent later.

The potential value of the scoring system in research was an implicit if unstated goal and was exploited at the outset by Apgar and her colleague,

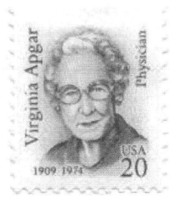

Figure 22.2 The 20-cent stamp honouring Virginia Apgar issued on 24 October 1994. (Photograph kindly supplied by Dr Alistair McKenzie.)

the New Zealand paediatrician LS James.[5] The first eight years of their clinical and experimental research demonstrated that during the first hours or days of life, there is a wide range of variation in many physiological measurements. It had been assumed that the respiratory and circulatory depression observed in infants with low scores were due to hypoxia, acidosis or a combination of both. To test this assumption, it became necessary to determine the oxygen content and hydrogen ion concentration (pH) of arterial blood. This Apgar obtained from the umbilical artery in an invasive procedure that at that time must have required considerable courage. '*She was the first person to catheterize the umbilical artery in a newborn infant,*' Dr James wrote in some awe, '*and undoubtedly the whole area of newborn intensive care would not be where it is today were it not for Virginia*'.[6] Umbilical artery catheterization has become standard procedure in the study of neonatal physiology, and its introduction represented an important step in the origins of the new field of neonatology.

As anticipated, the newborn babies with low Apgar Scores suffered hypoxia and acidosis – but this was more severe than anticipated. Even infants with high scores were found to have a low oxygen content and elevated hydrogen ion concentration (lower pH), reflecting a degree of asphyxia subsequently recognized as a normal physiological disturbance of the birth process. Their findings have been confirmed by subsequent investigators, and it was thought that blood gas analysis would make the Apgar Score obsolete. A *Lancet* editorial in 1989 stated that '*The Apgar*

Score has served its purpose, and should now be pensioned off.[7] This has not happened. Indeed, in the most recent research findings, published in the *New England Journal of Medicine*, the Apgar Score was found to be many times more accurate than umbilical artery acidosis in predicting the risk of neonatal death, from which the investigators concluded that *'the Apgar scoring system remains as relevant for the prediction of neonatal survival today as it was almost 50 years ago'*.[8] An accompanying editorial concluded that *'Its application at one minute of age accomplishes* [her] *goal of focussing attention on the condition of the infant immediately after birth'* and the five-minute score *'is still valid as a rapid method for assessing the effectiveness of resuscitative efforts and the vitality of the infant'*.[9]

Apgar's contributions to medicine were not limited to the care of the newborn and she had a wide range of other interests (Figure 22.3). In 1959, she obtained a Master's Degree in Public Health from the Johns Hopkins School of Medicine. She joined the staff of the National Foundation March of Dimes as Vice-President for Medical Affairs and Head of the Division of Congenital Malformations at a critical period

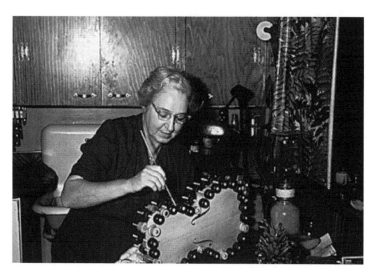

Figure 22.3 Virginia Apgar not only collected stamps, but was also a keen musician and made musical instruments. At the stamp dedication ceremony, a group of physicians/musicians called the Apgar String Quartet played some of her favourite music on instruments she had crafted herself. (Reproduced with the kind permission of Dr Selma Calmes.)

when the Foundation's resources were being diverted from poliomyelitis to the problem of birth defects. There, as Director of Research, she helped fund research into the genetic, infectious and environmental causes of birth defects. She spent her final years attempting to educate the public in the need for early detection of birth defects, and at the time of her death in 1974 at age 65, she was commuting from her Foundation job in New York to study genetics at Johns Hopkins in Baltimore.

References

1. Calmes SH. Virginia Apgar, M.D.: At the forefront of obstetric anesthesia. *American Society of Anesthesiology Newsletter* 1992;**56**:9–12.
2. Apgar V. A proposal for a new method of evaluation of the newborn infant. *Anesthesia and Analgesia* 1953;**32**:260–67.
3. Feinstein AR. Multi-item 'Instruments' vs Virginia Apgar's Principles of Clinimetrics. *Archives of Internal Medicine* 1999;**159**:125–8.
4. Apgar V. The Newborn (Apgar) Scoring System. Reflections and advice. *Pediatric Clinics of North America* 1966;**13**:645–50.
5. Apgar V, James LS. Further observations on the Newborn Scoring System. *American Journal of Diseases of Childhood* 1962;**194**:419–28.
6. James LS. Fond memories of Virginia Apgar. *Pediatrics* 1975;**55**:1–4.
7. Anonymous. Is the Apgar Score outmoded? *Lancet* 1989;**i**:591–2.
8. Casey B, McIntire DD, Leveno KJ. The continuing value of the Apgar score for the assessment of newborn infants. *New England Journal of Medicine* 2001;**344**:467–71.
9. Papik L-A. The Apgar score in the 21st century. *New England Journal of Medicine* 2001;**344**:519–20.

Part 5

Anaesthesia yesterday, today and tomorrow

23 Anaesthesia yesterday, today and tomorrow

During the last half-century, anaesthesia has been responsible for major changes in medical practice, and has become a scientific discipline in its own right. Today anaesthesia is one of the largest specialities in the UK National Health Service (NHS), but it faces two major problems: the impact of the European Working Time Directive on clinical services and training and the disintegration of the academic base that is essential for the future development of the subject.

In 1954, I (KS) was a junior anaesthetist at University College Hospital, London, and was awarded a Travelling Scholarship to enable me to visit departments of anaesthesia overseas. I decided to combine the travel with a year's Fellowship at the Massachusetts General Hospital, Boston. This hospital was chosen partly because of its known academic excellence, but also because there was a historical link between the two hospitals: the first ether anaesthetics for a surgical operation were administered in Boston on 16 October 1846 and in London on 21 December 1846. At the time of my visit, the Chairman and Henry Isaiah Dorr Professor of Anesthesia in Boston was HK Beecher, and his First Assistant was my collaborator on this book, JP Bunker. The Boston department had an international reputation for research in anaesthesia and the pharmacology of analgesic drugs, and the experience gained there, together with visits to over 40 Canadian and US departments, proved to be a turning point in my professional career.

There were many differences between the two institutions, but none greater than in the practice of anaesthesia.[1] In the UK, anaesthetics were only administered by doctors and speciality training lasted for six to eight years. In the USA, however, over 45% of anaesthetics were given by nurse–anesthetists who had trained in anaesthesia for two to three years after qualifying as nurses. Since the speciality training period for anesthesiologists was similar, surgeons treated them like nurses and dictated both the choice of anaesthetic and all perioperative therapy. Not surprisingly, the low status did not encourage junior doctors to enter the speciality, so anesthesiologists were in short supply.

This difference in practice had been established in the second half of the 19th century. In the UK, physicians such as John Snow and Joseph Clover had devoted much of their time to the practice of anaesthesia, but in the USA, surgeons had delegated the responsibility for administering anaesthesia to nurses; they believed that a nurse practising anaesthesia full-time would provide a better service than that offered by a doctor who only gave occasional anaesthetics. Nurse–anesthetists have continued to make a major contribution, both in the US Armed Forces and in civilian practice. Most work as part of anesthesiologist-led teams, but a significant number practise autonomously.

According to the American Association of Nurse Anesthetists, the first documented nurse–anesthetist was Sister Mary Bernard, a Catholic nun who worked in Erie, Pennsylvania, in 1887.[2] The Mayo brothers were quick to realise the value of anesthetic nurses, and Alice Magaw worked at St Mary's Hospital in Rochester, Minnesota, from 1889, soon becoming a legend in her time. The employment of nurse–anesthetists spread rapidly in the early 20th century, despite the campaign conducted by Francis McMechan and many other anesthesiologists who were strongly opposed to their employment. Some doctors have argued that their existence demeans the status of the anesthesiologist, while others have maintained that the anaesthetic service could not be maintained without them. The American Association of Nurse Anesthetists points out that nurse–anesthetists (40% of whom are male) undergo a rigorous two-year training programme and that they are re-certified every two years. It claims that Certified Registered Nurse Anesthetists currently administer about 65% of the 20–25 million anaesthetics administered annually in the USA.

While anaesthesia is one of the largest specialties in the UK, it has by far the lowest number of Consultants per 100 000 population (4.6 in the UK versus 10.8 in 17 European countries).[3] In calling attention to acute shortages in medically trained anaesthetists, it was suggested in a 1997 report by the Audit Commission that:

> 'The most fundamental way to reduce demands for more doctors substantially would be to adopt the anaesthesia system used in many other countries ... including much of Europe and the United States – that is, allowing non-medically qualified staff to maintain anaesthesia under the direct supervision of doctors. ... Such mid-

*level practitioners are frequently called "nurse anaesthetists"
although they do not have to come from a nursing background'.*[4]

The Audit Commission did not explicitly recommend the introduction of
non-medically qualified anaesthetists, but it did recommend study. The
careful wording of their recommendation deserves to be quoted in full:

*'Sponsor research on whether the demand for doctors can be
reduced, and the best use made of consultants' time, by allowing
others who are appropriately trained to monitor/maintain
anaesthesia without a medically qualified anaesthetist
continuously present in the operating room – for example, via
carefully controlled pilot schemes'.*[5]

The key to the nurse or 'non-medically qualified' anaesthetist problem is
the amount of medical knowledge required to provide safe anaesthesia.
Undoubtedly, the majority of fit patients undergoing routine surgery can be
anaesthetized safely by such practitioners. Their practice can be based on
established guidelines, and with careful training they can develop the
necessary technical skills for safe practice. The problems arise when they
have to anaesthetize a patient with severe pre-existing medical disease, or
when there is a complication of the surgery or anaesthesia that requires in-
depth medical knowledge for diagnosis and treatment. Nurse–anaesthetists
have practised with varying degrees of medical supervision in most
European countries for many years, and there is little evidence that their
use has resulted in a an increased mortality due to anaesthesia.[6] In Europe,
only Belgium and the UK have relied entirely on physician-based
anaesthesia, but, in the last few years, experimental training schemes for
non-medical graduates have been introduced into the UK in response to the
recommendations of the Audit Commission and recent government
initiatives. Many anaesthetists in the UK feel that the introduction of such
a grade will reduce the status of the anaesthetist, but others argue that there
are insufficient doctors to staff the NHS, and that it is better to have
properly trained non-medical personnel performing clearly defined tasks
than to have a breakdown of the service. The protagonists argue that, in
other specialities, nurses and other non-medical personnel are now
performing many tasks that were previously carried out by doctors and
that, in future, non-medical personnel must be used wherever they can
contribute usefully to the service.[7,8]

The staffing crisis

This raises the question of why there are not enough anaesthetists to fulfil
the service requirements. During the last 50 years, there has been a

continuous increase in the number of doctors practising anaesthesia in the UK. In the 1970s, there were about 1200 Consultants, 700 clinical assistants and an equal number of trainees,[9] but today there are more than 5000 Consultants (over a quarter being women), over 1200 non-career grade anaesthetists, and about 3500 doctors in training. There are a number of reasons for this expansion. First, there has been an increase in the number and range of surgical operations performed. For example, the specialities of open-heart surgery, transplant surgery, microsurgery and major arterial surgery were only just opening up in the 1960s, but now surgeons are operating on more patients who require skilled anaesthesia for prolonged periods. In addition, the increasing use of minimally invasive methods of surgery using telescopes and TV screens often increases the duration of the operation. Second, anaesthesia or sedation is now required for an increasing number of medical and radiological investigations, and for the rapidly expanding field of day-case surgery. Third, many anaesthetists have taken on extra responsibilities outside the operating theatre; anaesthetists now play a major role in hospital management, teaching, intensive care, resuscitation, accident and emergency medicine, the transport of seriously ill patients, and the treatment of acute and chronic pain.

The current crisis is, however, due mainly to the recent introduction of the European Working Time Directive that limits the number of hours a doctor can work. While accepting that the excessive workload, long hours and sleep deprivation that characterized medical practice in the 20th century are no longer acceptable, it must be noted that there are already concerns that the limit on working hours is compromising training and that continuity of patient care is suffering.[10–12] While training can be made more efficient by improving teaching methods and by using patient simulators and other aids to learning, there is no doubt that extensive graded experience in the clinical environment is an essential component of medical education. This is a serious problem that will be difficult to resolve.

Academic departments

The other major problem that is now being addressed in the UK is the decline in the number and quality of academic departments of anaesthesia. As we have seen, the first such department was created at Oxford in 1937, and in the postwar period many new academic departments of anaesthesia were developed.[13] Anaesthetists working in academic departments spent up to half of the working week in the operating theatre, intensive care unit or pain clinic, and the rest in teaching or research. Although the teaching of medical students or junior anaesthetists in the operating theatre or intensive care unit was shared with NHS Consultants, members of the academic staff also played a major role in the teaching of basic science to anaesthetists. These activities left little time for research. But whereas research projects in the 20th century were usually closely related to clinical problems, and could therefore often be integrated with clinical practice, today's research is concerned with more fundamental problems. These demand a higher degree of scientific expertise, more expensive equipment and a greater time commitment. Major research projects today involve collaboration between several different disciplines, and this again is difficult to achieve with limited funds and heavy clinical commitments. The problem is now being tackled on many fronts: the Royal College of Anaesthetists has formulated a National Strategy to tackle the problem,[14] but this has to be related to other major changes such as those proposed in the Walpole Report on Modernising Medical Careers.[15] It is a daunting task, but one that must be tackled expeditiously if anaesthesia is to continue to develop as a viable and forward-looking speciality.[16]

But anaesthetists have shown that they can face up to problems and that they are great facilitators. Over the last century and a half, they have made major advances in perioperative care and in the practice of acute medicine, and they have led the field in postgraduate education and in safe practice. If such progress can be maintained, anaesthesia should continue to make significant contributions to the practice of medicine.

References

1. Sykes MK. The American approach to anaesthesia. *British Medical Journal* 1956;**i**:1148–50.
2. American Association of Nurse Anesthetists website 15 November 2005.
3. Rolly G, MacRae WR, Blunnie WP, Dupont M, Scherpereel P. Anaesthesiological manpower in Europe. *European Journal of Anaesthesiology* 1996;**13**:325–32.
4. *Anaesthesia under Examination*. London: Audit Commission, 1997: 100.
5. Ibid: 104.
6. Smith AF, Kane M, Milne R. Comparative effectiveness and safety of physician and nurse anaesthetists: a narrative systematic review. *British Journal of Anaesthesia* 2004;**93**:540–5.
7. Kane M, Smith AF. An American tale – professional conflicts in anaesthesia in the United States: implications for the United Kingdom. *Anaesthesia* 2004;**59**:793–802.
8. Smith AF. Editorial. Anaesthetic practitioners in the UK: promise, perils and psychology. *Anaesthesia* 2005;**60**:1055–8.
9. Sykes MK. The staffing problem and its possible solutions. *Anaesthesia* 1973;**28**:364–72.

10. Greaves JD. Editorial: Training time and consultant practice. *British Journal of Anaesthesia* 2005;**95**:581–3.
11. Underwood SM, McIndoe AK. Influence of changing work patterns on training in anaesthesia: an analysis of activity in a UK teaching hospital from 1996–2004. *British Journal of Anaesthesia* 2005;**95**:616–21.
12. Spargo PM. UK anaesthetic training and the law of unintended consequences. Cause for concern? *Anaesthesia* 2005;**60**:319–22.
13. Nunn JF. Development of academic anaesthesia in the UK up to the end of 1998. *British Journal of Anaesthesia* 1999;**83**:916–32.
14. The Royal College of Anaesthetists. *A National Strategy for Academic Anaesthesia*, 2005. Available from www.rcoa.ac.uk.
15. *Medically- and Dentally-Qualified Academic Staff – Recommendations for Training the Researchers and Educators of the Future. Report of the Academic Careers Sub-Committee of Modernising Medical Careers and the UK Clinical Research Collaboration (The Walport Report)*. March 2005.
16. Pandit JJ. Editorial I. The national strategy for academic anaesthesia. A personal view of its implications for our speciality. *British Journal of Anaesthesia* 2006;**96**:411–14.

Index

Suffix 'n' refers to footnote.

Errata

Corrected text appears in **bold**; p.= page, l.= line, Fig. = figure. Line counts include headings.

p. 31, l. 5: …stimulators **and ultrasound probes** has…

p. 39, l. 14: **four of whose sons had died from the "summer disease"**, described how…

p. 39, l. 16: airway **when the larynx was obstructed in diphtheria**.

p. 55, l. 16: **1917**, the chair was established…

p. 63, Fig. 4.5 caption: John Silas Lundy (189**4**–1973),

p. 69, l. 2:. .Model T Ford **in the UK** and was selling. . .

p. 69, l. 22: St Thoma**s'** Hospital…

p. 81, Fig. 5.12 caption: Alexander Crampton Smith (1965–7**9**); Sir Keith Sykes (198**0**–91);

p. 83, l. 19: opportunity was **later** taken to change the…

p. 133, l. 6: rate of 8**4**% in the group given the traditional…

p. 133, l. 8: was subsequently reduced to **36%**. . .

p. 143, Fig. 10.5 caption: T Cecil Gray (1913–**2008**),

p. 153, l. 3 *et seq:* HWC Griffith**s** and John Gillies…

p. 162, l. 8: and of these 27 had died**,** a mortality rate of **nearly 90%**.

p. 162, l. 16: of the epidemic, **Henry Cai** Alexander Lassen…

p. 162, l. 17: Blegdam **Hospital for Infectious Diseases** (Figure 12.3)…

p. 164, l. 2: Morgens Bjørneboe, had travelled…

p. 164, l. 11: Frits Neukirch…

p. 164, Fig. 12.4: techniques for treating respiratory paralysis **in poliomyelitis**.

p. 165, l. 9: Ibsen had spent **a year** at the Massachusetts…

p. 174, l. 18: Norlander **and his colleagues**, described how…

p. 177, l. 17 from bottom: Hammersmith Hospital, **London,** doctors…

p. 185, l. 23: S. Andersen **in the mid-1930s**.

p. 185, l. 3 from bottom: **V Ray** Bennett.

p. 210, l. 8 from bottom: by William **Tossach** in 1732,

Index

Printed and bound by CPI Group (UK) Ltd, Croydon, CR0 4YY

23/10/2024

01777665-0001